COLON & RECTAL CANCER

From Diagnosis to Treatment

Third Edition

PAUL RUGGIERI, M.D.
ARTI LAKHANI, M.D.

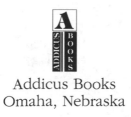

Addicus Books
Omaha, Nebraska

An Addicus Nonfiction Book

ISBN: 978-1-943886-83-8
Illustrations and typography by Jack Kusler

This book is not intended to be a substitute for a physician, nor do the authors intend to give advice contrary to that of an attending physician.

Library of Congress Cataloging-in-Publication Data
Names: Ruggieri, Paul, 1959- author. | Lakhani, Arti, 1982- author.
Title: Colon & rectal cancer : from diagnosis to treatment / Paul Ruggieri, M.D., Arti Lakhani, M.D.
Other titles: Colon and rectal cancer
Description: Third edition. | Omaha, Nebraska : Addicus Books, [2018] | Includes index.
Identifiers: LCCN 2018038276 (print) | LCCN 2018038655 (ebook) | ISBN 9781943886906 (pdf) | ISBN 9781943886999 (kdl) | ISBN 9781943886982 (epub) | ISBN 9781943886838 (paperback)
Subjects: LCSH: Colon (Anatomy)—Cancer. | Rectum—Cancer. | BISAC: MEDICAL / Oncology. | MEDICAL / Diseases.
Classification: LCC RC280.C6 (ebook) | LCC RC280.C6 R84 2018 (print) | DDC 616.99/4347—dc23
LC record available at https://lccn.loc.gov/2018038276

Addicus Books, Inc.
P.O. Box 45327
Omaha, Nebraska 68145
www.AddicusBooks.com

Printed in the United States of America
10 9 8 7 6 5 4 3 2 1

Contents

Acknowledgments

I would first like to thank all my patients, past and present, for the privilege of being involved in their care. I would also like to acknowledge my patients' family members. Their love, understanding, and support are so vital to a loved one's recovery.

I would like to thank Christine Gillespie, R.N., both for her care of my colorectal cancer patients and for her input in this book. I wish to thank Diane Peckham, R.N., retired certified wound, ostomy, and continence nurse, for her expertise on the care of a colostomy and for introducing me to my future wife.

I wish to thank radiation oncologist Carol Kornmehl, M.D., author of *The Best News about Radiation Therapy*, for her contribution to the chapter on radiation therapy. I would also like to thank Mark Pool, M.D., Laboratory Medical Director at Riverside Medical Center, Kankakee, Illinois, for his help in the development of this book.

This book would not have been possible without the efforts of all those involved at Addicus Books. I especially thank Rod Colvin for his uncompromising focus and drive for perfection. I also express my appreciation to Jack Kusler for his illustrations and design work.

Finally, I would like to thank Larry Connors for his inspiration, and my parents for their courage and support.

Paul Ruggieri, M.D.

First and foremost, I'd like to thank my patients for helping to make this book possible; your strength and courage humbles me. I learn from you every day, and this knowledge has helped me become a better physician. I would also like to thank my partners and my colleagues for their support. I have seen how you treat your patients and ease their ailments. Many of your ideas have gone into this book.

This book would not have been possible without the editorial support of Mary Meyer, who shares my dedication and passion to improve the quality of life of cancer patients.

Finally, many thanks to Jack Kusler, Rod Colvin, and everyone at Addicus Books for their desire to educate and bring comfort to patients. I'm proud to be part of educating and empowering patients so they can take an active role in their own health care.

Arti Lakhani, M.D.

Introduction

Has your life suddenly been interrupted by an unexpected diagnosis of colon or rectal cancer? Or, has someone close to you just been diagnosed with the disease? If so, your first reaction may be shock, denial, or anger. It doesn't seem fair that you're suddenly forced to come face-to-face with a life-threatening disease. You may be thinking, Why me? Why my family? Your reactions and feelings are normal and understandable. It may be of comfort to know that you are not alone.

Unfortunately, cancer affects nearly everyone directly or indirectly. If you or an immediate family member has not been diagnosed with it, you probably know someone who has. This is especially true of colorectal cancer. Colon cancer is the second most common cancer in the United States, and the third leading cause of cancer deaths in the United States.

Our goal in writing this book is to provide you with some peace of mind by answering those pressing questions that arise with a diagnosis of cancer. It is our hope that this book will serve as your guide as you make the journey through treatment.

1 COLORECTAL CANCER: AN OVERVIEW

It seems nothing can prepare us for a diagnosis of cancer. Being told you have cancer can bring on a flood of emotions—shock, fear, and confusion. At first, it may be difficult to comprehend the fact that you have cancer. In addition to coming to grips with the diagnosis, you're faced with undergoing medical tests and a series of treatments, all of which you probably know little about. It can be a stressful time for you, your family, and friends.

The term *colorectal cancer* actually refers to two diseases. Colon cancer is cancer found in the tissues of the colon, and rectal cancer forms in the tissues of the rectum. Both cancers have the same characteristics and the same risk factors. In some cases, they are treated the same way, while at other times the treatments are different.

Colorectal Cancer Statistics

Not counting skin cancer, colon cancer is the third most commonly diagnosed cancer in the United States. It affects approximately 96,000 Americans each year, according to the American Cancer Society. Rectal cancer is less common than colon cancer, affecting nearly 40,000 people annually. Both cancers are curable if detected early. And, thanks to improved treatments and greater public awareness about preventive screening, death rates from colorectal cancer have been dropping over the last twenty years.

1

Colorectal Cancer in the United States

Colon cancer cases diagnosed annually:
- Men: 47,000
- Women: 47,000

Rectal cancer cases diagnosed annually:
- Men: 23,000
- Women: 16,000

Approximately 72 percent of cases are colon cancer.

Approximately 28 percent of cases are rectal cancer.

Lifetime chances of developing colorectal cancer: 1 in 20

American Cancer Society

Anatomy and Function of the Colon and Rectum

Before discussing colorectal cancer and how it develops, let's first take a brief look at the anatomy of the colon and rectum. The colon and rectum are important parts of your *gastrointestinal (GI) tract.* This tract includes your mouth, *esophagus*, stomach, small intestine, colon (large intestine), rectum, and anus. This system takes in food, digests it, absorbs nutrients, and excretes waste.

The primary job of the colon is to manage and remove solid waste. When you eat, food spends several hours in the stomach being digested. Once the nutrients are absorbed in the small intestine, any remaining liquid enters the *colon,* which is also called the *large bowel.*

By the time the liquid enters the first part of the colon, it contains no nutrients and is pure waste product. This waste liquid is slowly propelled toward the rectum. Over a four- to six-hour period, the cells in the colon absorb remaining water from the waste material. The colon can absorb nearly two gallons of water a day. The end product is the solid waste, or feces.

The rectum's primary function is to store processed fecal material before it is excreted from the body. Once

Frontal View of Colon

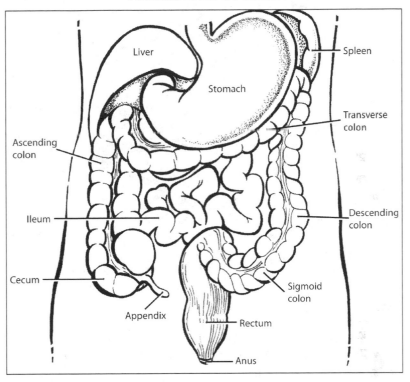

there is enough fecal material in the rectum, sensory nerves tell the brain it is time to have a bowel movement.

The Colon

The colon is a hollow, tubelike organ that is five to six feet long and up to five inches in diameter. It sits in the abdominal cavity and is divided into segments. The first segment is the *cecum,* which is a pouch that receives waste material from the small intestine. The next segment is the *right (ascending) colon,* located on the right side of the abdomen. The *transverse colon* crosses over the midsection of the abdomen. The *left (descending) colon* is on the left side of the abdominal cavity. The left colon leads into the *sigmoid colon,* an S-shaped section that

3

connects to the rectum. The rectum is a muscular tube, the last six to ten inches of the colon, and it exits into the anus.

The colon itself has four layers of tissue. The innermost layer, the *mucosa*, is in direct contact with fecal material moving through the colon and is responsible for much of the colon's function. The thin mucosa is composed of specialized cells that are in a constant state of flux, continually dying, sloughing off, and being replaced with new cells. The layer under the mucosa is the *submucosa*. It's a specialized layer of cells that helps support the mucosa.

The next layer of tissue is the *muscularis propria.* The muscle cells in this layer give strength to the colon wall and cause the contractions that push fecal material along the colon. The outermost layer of tissue is the *serosa.* The serosal cells add more support to the colon wall and act as a barrier, protecting the colon from any outside invading disease.

The Rectum

The rectum, the last six to ten inches of the colon, connects the colon to the anus. Unlike the rest of the colon, the walls of the rectum are primarily composed of muscle cells that propel the fecal material out of the body.

The last part of the digestive system is the anus. It is a canal, about two inches long, that contains sphincter muscles; it's the job of these muscles to hold in waste material until you're ready to have a bowel movement.

How Colorectal Cancer Develops

Colorectal cancer usually develops from *polyps*, which are small, abnormal growths that can occur anywhere along the gastrointestinal tract. Polyps are common in the colon and rectum; in fact, as many as 50 percent of the U.S. population has polyps in the colon and/or rectum. Polyps occur more frequently in people over age fifty;

they are caused by changes in the cells lining the inside of the colon and grow slowly over a period of ten to fifteen years. Cancer is an overgrowth of these abnormal cells and, sometimes, polyps start growing uncontrollably. Most people have no idea a tumor is growing inside their colon or rectum unless they go for routine tests or start to experience symptoms such as pain or bleeding.

Types of Polyps

Colorectal polyps may be benign or malignant (cancerous). Fortunately, most polyps are benign. Only about 1 percent of polyps that are removed prove to be cancerous. Still, it's important to know that some polyps can turn into cancer if not removed.

Benign Polyps

Polyps referred to as benign are noncancerous. Several types of benign polyps may occur in the colon. The polyps are defined by their size and the appearance of their cells under the microscope.

- *Hyperplastic.* About 90 percent of all polyps are hyperplastic polyps. They are small, about the size of a pea, and consist of a dense cluster of normal cells with no microscopic abnormalities. They are totally benign, with no potential to become cancerous.

- *Inflammatory.* This type of benign polyp, also small, is made up of inflamed cells commonly associated with inflammatory diseases of the colon, including ulcerative colitis and Crohn's disease.

- *Hamartoma.* This type of small, benign polyp is found in patients with genetically inherited polyp syndromes. (*See* discussion of these syndromes later in this chapter.) These polyps are frequently numerous and scattered throughout the colon.

Polyp Shapes

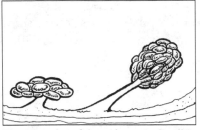 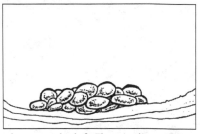

The examples of the polyps on a "stalk" are shown on the left. These polyps are less likely to be cancerous. The polyps on the right are broad based, or sessile, and are more likely to be cancerous.

Precancerous Polyps

A polyp can also be labeled *precancerous*. This means the growth contains suspicious-looking cells when viewed under the microscope, but these cells do not yet meet the criteria to be called malignant. If precancerous cells are not removed or treated, they can develop into cancer that can spread. These polyps are divided into three categories.

- *Tubular.* This type of polyp may be found anywhere in the colon. Most are about one-fourth inch in diameter but may grow to three-fourths inch. They are made up of cells that are tubular in shape. Tubular polyps are generally considered premalignant with a 5 percent chance of becoming cancerous if not removed.

- *Tubulovillous.* This type of polyp typically grows to about one-half inch in diameter and has a cluster of fingerlike projections. These polyps have a higher potential—20 percent—to turn into cancer.

- *Villous.* These premalignant polyps are often found in the rectal area; they can grow to one to two inches in diameter. Villous polyps have the greatest potential—up to a 40 percent chance—to become malignant.

Cancerous Polyps

When a polyp is found to be cancerous, the cancer may be classified as *carcinoma in situ* or as *adenocarcinoma*.

- *Carcinoma in situ.* These polyps contain cancer cells that are at the beginning of their life cycle. The malignant cells are contained within the polyp and do not spread to other organs.

- *Adenocarcinoma.* These cancerous polyps have the potential to spread outside the polyp to other organs. This type of cancer is the most common form of colorectal cancer, making up nearly 96 percent of all cases.

Characteristics of Cancerous Polyps

Several factors influence whether a colorectal polyp is malignant. These factors include the size of the polyp, its shape, location in the colon, and the presence or absence of microscopic changes to the DNA, the cell's blueprint for growth.

Size

The larger the polyp, the greater the chance of it being cancerous. For instance, a polyp less than one-half inch in diameter has a less than 10 percent chance of being cancerous. However, polyps more than one inch in diameter can have a 20 to 30 percent chance of being cancerous. It is important to remove polyps early so they cannot grow to sizes that increase the potential for cancer.

Shape

The general shape of a colorectal polyp also influences the potential of it being cancerous. Polyps that are located on a "stalk," with the stalk attached to the inner lining of the colon wall, are easily removed and less likely to be cancerous. However, polyps that are very broad based are more difficult to remove and more likely to be cancerous. Broad-based polyps are called *sessile polyps.*

Location

The location of a polyp is also important. Cancerous polyps are more commonly found in the sigmoid colon and rectum than in other parts of the colon. It has been estimated that more than 50 percent of cancerous polyps are located in the sigmoid colon and rectum; the sigmoid is the part of the large intestine that is closest to the rectum and anus.

Dysplasia

Dysplasia is the medical term used to describe the genetic mutations (abnormalities) observed in the DNA of polyp cells. When cells are dysplastic their centers (*nuclei*) are misshapen. The more dysplastic changes, the greater the chance of finding cancer cells. Dysplastic changes can lead to cancerous tumors.

Symptoms of Colorectal Cancer

Early on, the symptoms of colorectal cancer often go unnoticed. You may feel fine, with no indication of any problem. Fortunately, routine screening often leads to the detection of colorectal cancer even when you have no symptoms.

By the time symptoms are obvious, colorectal cancer has often progressed. Unfortunately, many people ignore the signs and do not report them to their doctor. Some people do not realize that a change in bowel habits or blood in the stool may be a sign of cancer. Other people are embarrassed to talk about such symptoms. However, ignoring such symptoms may delay the early diagnosis of a potentially curable cancer.

Symptoms of Colorectal Cancer

- Fatigue caused by iron deficiency anemia
- Change in bowel habits
- Rectal bleeding
- Chronic abdominal pain, bloating, or fullness
- Painful urge to have a bowel movement
- Decreased appetite or unintended weight loss

Fatigue

Fatigue has many causes and is not always a symptom of colorectal cancer. However, when fatigue is caused by iron deficiency anemia, it may be a symptom of colorectal cancer. This anemia is caused by the body's not receiving enough iron to produce healthy *red blood cells*, which carry oxygen to the body's other cells. Such anemia could be the result of the slow, progressive loss of blood caused by a tumor. You may not notice the anemia right away, but it can lead to noticeable symptoms such as fatigue, pale appearance, dizziness, or shortness of breath during physical activity.

Change in Bowel Habits

A common early-warning symptom of colorectal cancer is a subtle change in your bowel habits. Changes in your bowel pattern may include:

- Persistent loose stools
- Constipation
- Vague discomfort with bowel movements
- Changes in the shape of stools, such as pencil-thin stools
- A painful urge to have a bowel movement when it's not needed. This urge or feeling of incomplete evacuation of the bowels is known as *tenesmus*.

It may be caused by a tumor growing inside the rectum that takes up space and creates pressure.

Rectal Bleeding

Passing bright red or dark blood is another warning symptom of colorectal cancer. The bleeding may be coming from a polyp or a cancer. You may notice blood on toilet paper or blood mixed in with a bowel movement; if the blood is mixed with stool, it may be dark, almost black, in color.

Passing blood may occur without pain. You may not even notice it if the blood loss is subtle and occurs slowly. It is possible that rectal bleeding could be caused by a hemorrhoid; however, it's important to report any rectal bleeding to your physician.

Abdominal Pain or Bloating

Abdominal pain is not a common warning symptom for colorectal cancer during its early stages. However, if the disease has spread beyond the colon or rectal wall into other organs, abdominal cramping and pain may occur. Individuals with this type of abdominal pain usually describe it as a dull, nagging, intermittent pain that does not go away with the use of over-the-counter antacids. Unfortunately, many people ignore such pain until it starts to impact their everyday activities. If you have recurrent pain, do not attribute it to an upset stomach, stress, or food choices. If the cancer should cause a perforation in the colon, the pain will likely worsen and may require a visit to an emergency room.

Other times, people may not feel pain, but will report feeling full after eating very little. If cancer has spread to the inner lining of the abdominal cavity, an accumulation of fluid may result. This may cause bloating or rapid distension of the belly. Sometimes, people say they can feel a mass in their abdomen that was never there before.

If you experience any of these symptoms, see your doctor.

Decreased Appetite or Unintended Weight Loss

Some people with colorectal cancer complain of not having an appetite or of losing weight despite eating. It's possible that appetite could be affected by a tumor or fluid in the abdomen, causing you to feel full after eating very little. The reason that having cancer may cause weight loss is complex and not totally understood. It is believed that when you have cancer, the body releases destructive proteins, which leads to an increased metabolic rate that is too high for sustaining body weight. Your body may not be absorbing all the fat, protein, and carbohydrates from the food you eat. Or your body may be burning calories faster than normal. The result is weight loss.

Bacterial Infection

Sometimes, colorectal cancer will cause an abscess in the abdomen. Bacteria that reside in the colon can escape through the abscess and into the bloodstream. Having an infection in the bloodstream is a serious, life-threatening condition. It is referred to as *bacteremia,* or *sepsis.* Symptoms include chills, fever, drop in blood pressure, rapid heart rate, hyperventilation, light-headedness, and confusion. This condition requires emergency medical care.

Stroke-Like Symptoms

Symptoms similar to those of a stroke are rarely the first symptoms of colorectal cancer. However, it is possible that some colorectal cancers may go undetected until the cancer has spread to parts of the brain. Symptoms would include stroke-like symptoms, such as weakness or numbness in the face, arm, or leg. Other possible symptoms are blurred vision, slurred speech, and seizures.

Risk Factors for Colorectal Cancer

What are the risks for developing colorectal cancer? No one knows exactly what causes colorectal cancer. However, doctors think genetic changes, coupled with dietary and environmental factors, play a role in normal cells changing into cancerous cells.

The following risk factors increase the chances for developing colorectal cancer sometime in your life. Fortunately, some of the risks are related to lifestyle, and making changes in lifestyle can decrease your risk.

Family History

A family history of colorectal cancer is the most important risk factor. According to the National Cancer Institute, 25 percent of individuals diagnosed with colon cancer have a family history of the disease. Having someone in your family with colorectal cancer, particularly a parent or sibling, puts you at a much higher risk than someone without a family history of the disease. If a relative such as an aunt, uncle, or cousin has had colorectal cancer, the risk is lower, but still higher than for those with no family history of the disease.

Several genetically inherited syndromes may predispose you to developing early colorectal cancer. If you or a member of your family is diagnosed with one of these syndromes, you're at higher risk. Fortunately, most of these syndromes are rare. However, they can be deadly if not diagnosed and treated early.

Hereditary nonpolyposis colorectal cancer (HNPCC), also known as *Lynch syndrome,* accounts for about 5 percent of all colon cancers. It causes the formation of one to five potentially cancerous polyps in people in their thirties or forties; however, the polyps can also occur earlier, before age twenty. Individuals with this syndrome have an 80 percent chance of developing colon cancer at some point in their lives.

Families with this abnormal gene usually have three or more closely related family members who have been diagnosed with colorectal cancer, colon cancer affecting family members in two generations, and at least one family member who has been diagnosed with colorectal cancer before the age of fifty.

Familial adenomatous polyposis (FAP) is a rare, inherited disease that causes the formation of hundreds or even thousands of polyps along the gastrointestinal tract. These polyps typically form during the teenage years and, if left untreated, will nearly always turn cancerous by the time the person reaches his or her late thirties. This syndrome is mostly associated with polyps in the colon, but may affect other organs, such as the liver, thyroid gland, and brain.

Gardner's syndrome is another rare disease. A variation of FAP, it can cause hundreds of polyps in the colon or small intestine; it may also cause benign tumors in the skin, bone, or abdomen.

Turcot syndrom is a rare, inherited disorder in which multiple polyps form in the colon, causing an increased risk for colon cancer. There is also a risk of cancer developing in the brain.

Peutz-Jeghers syndrome is a condition marked by the development of freckles all over the body. Polyps, which may become malignant, form in the colon.

Cowden syndrome is a rare disorder that causes benign tumors in the skin and mucous membranes of the mouth and nose. However, polyps may form in the colon, increasing the risk for colon cancer.

Finally, there is also increasing evidence that a family history of uterine, breast, or ovarian cancer may increase the risk for colorectal cancer. Knowing your family history is important to understanding your risk and developing a screening plan with your doctor.

Age

Anyone at any age can develop colorectal cancer. However, more than 90 percent of the people diagnosed with colorectal cancer are over the age of fifty. The average age of people diagnosed with colorectal cancer is close to seventy. If you're under age forty and have no other risk factors, you're at very low risk for getting colorectal cancer. After age fifty, however, population studies show that your risk increases dramatically. That's why routine checkups and screening for most people should start at age fifty.

Medical History

If you have had colorectal polyps or have been treated for colorectal cancer in the past, you are at a much higher risk for redeveloping either disease in the future. Follow-up tests after you have been treated for colorectal cancer are critical.

Diet

What you eat affects your risk. A diet high in meat and saturated fats and low in fiber (the so-called Western diet) places you at greater risk for developing colorectal cancer.

This is evident in studies of Japanese immigrants to the United States. The incidence of colorectal cancer in Japan is much lower than in the United States. This is presumably due to the high-fiber, low-fat diet prevalent in Japan. However, when Japanese come to the United States and adopt a more Western diet, within two generations their risk of developing colorectal cancer is the same as that of Americans.

The risk stems from potential cancer-causing agents, or *carcinogens*, that can form when the body ingests fatty acids and cholesterol. When fatty foods are cooked and processed, saturated fatty acids and cholesterol are broken down into potential cancer-causing by-products. Over time, these carcinogens interact with the cells lining the

14

inside of the colon, damaging their DNA. The damaged (mutated) DNA can then greatly increase the potential of these cells to turn cancerous.

It is well known that a diet high in fiber can reduce the risk for many diseases affecting the colon, including cancer. Fiber is thought to trap or dilute the cancer-causing agents in our diet. Fiber also flushes out these agents quickly, decreasing the time they are in contact with the lining of the colon.

Inflammatory Bowel Diseases

Two *inflammatory bowel diseases* that affect the lining of the colon are associated with an increased risk of colorectal cancer over time. These diseases are *ulcerative colitis* and *Crohn's disease.*

Ulcerative colitis causes inflammation of the inner layer of colon cells and results in chronic pain, bleeding, and diarrhea. It can affect an isolated segment of the colon or the entire organ. The cause of ulcerative colitis is not known, and there is no effective medical cure. Surgery often is the only potential curative option, but it can't prevent the disease from coming back later in life. During the first ten years that a person has ulcerative colitis, the risk of developing colorectal cancer is low. However, after the first ten years, the risk increases 20 percent every ten years. Routine screening should begin after the initial diagnosis.

Crohn's disease also increases the risk for colorectal cancer. Like ulcerative colitis, Crohn's disease involves inflammation of the inner layer of the colon. It usually also involves other layers of the colon wall. Crohn's disease leads to abdominal pain, bleeding, infection, blockages, and diarrhea. The disease has no known cause, and treatment can be difficult. The longer a person lives with Crohn's disease, the greater the risk for developing colorectal cancer.

Smoking

Studies by the American Cancer Society show that prolonged smoking can significantly increase your risk of colorectal cancer. According to the data, if you have smoked for more than twenty years, your risk of dying from colorectal cancer increases 40 percent. Clearly, the more you smoke, the more you increase your risk of cancer. It is also evident that the younger you start smoking, the greater your risk. This is true for both men and women.

Obesity and Physical Inactivity

Several medical studies indicate that being overweight and physically inactive increases the risk for colorectal cancer. If you're very overweight—especially if you carry your excess weight around your waist—you're at even greater risk for colorectal cancer. Some research suggests that excess fat changes metabolism (how the body converts food to energy) in a way that increases the growth of cells in the colon.

People who don't get a minimum amount of exercise are also at increased risk for colorectal cancer. Studies suggest that exercise, including aerobic and strength training, may lower the risk for colorectal cancer. Exercise also has well-known benefits for the heart and lungs and helps control weight.

Exposure to Asbestos

Some studies show an increased risk of colorectal cancer for workers who have had contact with asbestos, the fibrous material once used in insulation for residential and commercial construction. The Agency for Toxic Substances and Disease Registry (ATSDR) agrees that some studies show a link between asbestos exposure and colorectal cancer; however, the agency says there is no definitive proof that exposure to asbestos causes colorectal cancer.

In Summary

We've discussed some of the potential causes of colon and rectal cancer along with symptoms. If you have these symptoms, you may have already undergone diagnostic testing. Or, perhaps you are scheduled for tests. The next chapter discusses the medical tests that are commonly used to diagnose colon and rectal cancer.

2 GETTING A DIAGNOSIS

Getting colorectal cancer diagnosed early might mean the difference between curing the cancer and discovering that the cancer has advanced. The five-year survival rate for people who are diagnosed and treated early is 90 percent.

It takes five to ten years for colon cancer to grow through the colon wall; hopefully this expanse of time will increase the likelihood that an individual will have a colon cancer screening test or seek medical attention for symptoms. Still, doctors cannot predict which cancers will spread. Some smaller tumors may, for reasons not fully known, release cancer cells into the bloodstream, allowing them to spread to other organs. Other times, tumors may grow to a large size but not spread.

About 37 percent of colorectal cancers are detected early, before any spread has occurred. However, approximately 37 percent of the time, the cancer has spread to surrounding tissues. In about 20 percent of cases, the cancer has spread to distant organs.

Medical History and Physical Examination

During a visit to your doctor, he or she will take a personal and medical history and ask you about your symptoms. The doctor will ask about any changes in your bowel habits, passing of blood, abdominal pain, weight loss, and/or decreased appetite. The doctor will also want to know if you have any family history of colorectal cancer, including which relatives may have had colon cancer and their ages at the time of diagnosis. A complete and accurate personal and family medical history can provide your doctor with important clues that can help diagnose your condition.

Your physician will also likely perform a thorough physical examination. He or she will observe whether you're pale, which can be a sign of anemia, a deficiency in red blood cells. The doctor will perform a digital exam of your rectum, checking for possible masses; the doctor will also examine your abdomen to detect any bloating or masses. However, if cancer is just starting, the doctor may not find anything abnormal during the initial exam.

Diagnostic Tests

If colorectal cancer is suspected, your physician will schedule you for diagnostic testing. He or she may do the initial testing and then may refer you to specialists for additional testing.

Fecal Occult Blood Test

The *fecal occult blood test (FOBT)* is used to find occult (hidden) blood in your feces. The screening involves placing a smear of stool on a card and applying a drop of a liquid chemical onto the feces. If a trace amount of blood is present in your stool, the card turns blue, a positive test result. Only 2 to 4 percent of patients tested will be found to have a positive test for fecal occult blood.

A positive FOBT result does *not* necessarily mean you have colorectal cancer. It means your doctor needs to perform additional tests to find the source of the blood. One negative aspect of the fecal occult blood test is its accuracy. The test is not very specific for the presence of colorectal cancer. There are many other diseases of the colon, including hemorrhoids, rectal ulcers, fissures,

Crohn's disease, ulcerative colitis, *diverticulosis*, polyps, and trauma from the exam itself that can cause you to have a positive test result. Despite not being very specific, the fecal occult blood test is simple, cost-effective, and helpful in beginning the process of detecting colorectal cancer.

Stool DNA Test

A newer test, the *stool DNA test* is similar to the fecal occult blood test, which looks for blood in the stool. However, the stool DNA test is used to check for both blood and abnormal genetic materials from polyps or cancer cells. Polyps and colon cancers are continually shedding DNA cells that will eventually show up in the stool.

The test is not invasive and requires no preparation to clean out the colon. It does require the collection of an entire stool sample. Typically, patients are given special kits for collecting the sample, which must reach the laboratory within twenty-four hours. This test is not used widely because of the need for the entire stool sample and because it is more expensive to test the DNA.

Colonoscopy

A *colonoscopy* is considered the best diagnostic test for colorectal cancer. It is the most effective way to evaluate the inside of your entire colon for the presence of polyps or cancer. Because the colonoscope has wire snares and biopsy forceps, a doctor can also remove any polyps that are found and can biopsy or even remove a tumor. Performed in an outpatient setting, at a hospital or surgery center, the procedure is performed by either a gastroenterologist or a general surgeon.

Your colon must be empty and clean before the procedure. This usually involves drinking a liquid laxative and avoiding solid foods the day before; you'll be allowed to drink only clear liquids. Before undergoing a colonoscopy, you'll be given light sedation since the procedure can cause some discomfort as the colonoscope is guided through the colon.

To perform the procedure, the physician gradually advances a flexible fiber-optic scope through the entire colon. Air inflates the colon so the doctor can have a clear view of the entire colon lining on a television monitor. The procedure takes approximately thirty minutes.

Afterward, you'll be taken to a recovery area and monitored by nurses until you're awake. You'll need to have someone take you to the procedure and pick you up afterward. Typically, before you leave, your doctor will let you know whether any polyps or tumors were detected. If either is found, laboratory tests will be performed on the tissues to determine whether cancer is present.

Colonoscopy is safe, but not totally risk free. Possible complications include bleeding after polyp removal, and perforation of the colon. Perforation of the colon is rare, occurring 0.2 to 0.4 percent of the time; this complication, however, does require emergency surgery to repair. In addition, potential adverse reactions to the intravenous sedation include nausea, vomiting, and temporary breathing distress.

About 10 to 20 percent of the time, the physician is unable to view the entire colon successfully. This may be a result of incomplete bowel cleansing the day before, or the doctor may not be able to navigate all the turns in the colon. When this occurs, a follow-up barium enema may be necessary to complete the examination.

Flexible Sigmoidoscopy

The *flexible sigmoidoscopy* is a test that allows a doctor to check for polyps or cancer in the lower part of the intestine, where nearly 50 percent of all colorectal cancer occurs.

The sigmoidoscope is a thin, flexible fiber-optic tube that contains a tiny camera at the tip. The tube, about

Colonoscopy

Sigmoidoscopy

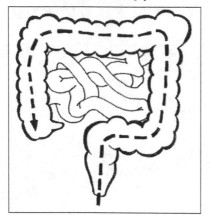
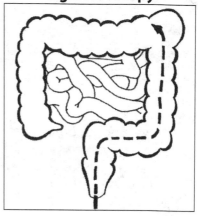

A colonoscopy is performed to examine the entire colon for polyps or cancer.

A sigmoidoscopy is performed to examine the lower portion of the colon.

thirty inches long, is connected to a television monitor, allowing the doctor to examine the last several feet of the colon (sigmoid colon) and the entire rectum. The procedure is carried out in the doctor's office and takes about ten minutes. No anesthesia is necessary since the procedure isn't painful. The procedure may be performed by your primary care doctor, an internist, a general surgeon, or a *gastroenterologist,* who is a physician trained in diagnosing and treating diseases of the colon.

During a sigmoidoscopy, as the scope is inserted into the anus and directed into the rectum, you'll feel a slight pressure sensation as air is pumped through the scope and into the colon. The air expands the inside of the colon so the doctor can examine the entire lining. If a polyp or tumor is discovered, it can be removed with the sigmoidoscope for laboratory examination.

If your doctor orders a sigmoidoscopy, you'll be instructed to give yourself an enema the night before the procedure to cleanse your bowels. You'll need to avoid food and beverages on the morning of the procedure;

however, your doctor will likely tell you it's okay to take medications with water.

The flexible sigmoidoscopy has several advantages: It can be performed in five to fifteen minutes in a doctor's office; it usually does not cause discomfort; and it carries less risk for complications than a colonoscopy.

The disadvantage is that since it is used to examine only the lower part of the colon, it can miss polyps and cancers in other parts of the colon. Studies have shown that if your screening flexible sigmoidoscopy is normal, there is up to a 3 percent chance you could still have a cancer in the side of your colon not reached by the sigmoidscope.

Possible complications of sigmoidoscopy include perforation of the colon or rectum by the scope. These complications are rare, however, occurring in only 1 out of 10,000 procedures. However, if a perforation does occur, emergency surgery is needed to repair the perforation.

Computerized Tomography (CT) Colonography

Another test used to examine the colon is the *computerized tomography (CT) colonography*, also known as a *virtual colonoscopy*. In this procedure, a scope is not inserted through the rectum. Instead, you are placed inside a sophisticated computerized tomography (CT or CAT) scanner; the scan provides detailed two- and three-dimensional images of your colon.

The procedure has several advantages: It is less invasive and less uncomfortable than a standard colonoscopy; it can be done in about ten minutes; and it does not require sedation. However, a rubber tube used to insert air into the colon to expand it is still needed. The bowel-cleansing preparation is also the same as for other tests using a scope. If a polyp is found on a virtual colonoscopy, you will still need a standard colonoscopy to have it removed.

Double-Contrast Barium Enema

If your doctor decides your entire colon needs evaluation, he or she may order a *double-contrast barium enema*, which may be done at the same time as a flexible sigmoidoscopy. During the procedure, air and barium, a white liquid (contrast), are injected into the bowels through a tube that is inserted in the rectum. Several X-rays are taken and then read by a *radiologist*, a doctor trained in reading X-rays. The procedure takes an hour and is performed on an outpatient basis in the radiology department of a hospital or surgery center. Although this test isn't painful, most people experience a sensation of pressure, which may be uncomfortable.

If your doctor orders this test, you will be given advance instructions. The day before the procedure, you will be asked to drink a substance that cleanses the inside of your colon.

The double-contrast barium enema is not used as often as it once was. Although it is accurate enough to identify most large polyps and cancerous colorectal tumors, it can miss small polyps less than one inch in size.

Other Blood Tests

There is no specific blood test for colon cancer; however, your doctor may order blood tests if he or she suspects the presence of a colorectal cancer. A *complete blood count (CBC)* is a test performed to evaluate your red blood cell count. This test checks your hemoglobin and hematocrit. *Hemoglobin* is related to the amount of iron circulating in your blood. *Hematocrit* refers to the percentage of red blood cells in your total blood volume. If both values are lower than normal, you have a condition called *anemia.*

Anemia can be caused by slowly losing blood over several months from a growing colorectal cancer. However, having anemia does not necessarily mean you have colorectal cancer. Anemia can be caused by a number of other health problems.

A word of caution about blood tests: If you have an abnormal blood test, remember that abnormal test results alone do *not* necessarily mean you have colorectal cancer. Your doctor will need to put these results in perspective with your symptoms and the results of other tests before being able to determine whether cancer is present.

Other Diagnostic Tests

Your doctor may order other tests if he or she suspects colorectal cancer. Many times, these tests are ordered to evaluate whether a newly diagnosed cancer has spread to other parts of the body. The tests are also ordered in anticipation of treatment, such as surgery or chemotherapy. The tests are performed in an outpatient setting; they are noninvasive and involve no discomfort.

Computerized Axial Tomography (CAT) Scan

A *computerized axial tomography scan* is commonly referred to as a *CAT scan* or a *CT scan*. This type of scan uses special X-ray equipment and computers to take a series of detailed photos of the body's internal organs, tissues, bones, and blood vessels. If you have been diagnosed with colorectal cancer, the scan can help determine whether the cancer is confined to the colon or whether it may have spread.

For this test, you lie on an examination table that moves slowly through the scanning machine, which has a large hole in the middle of it. The machine takes pictures that are similar to X-rays; however, the images produced by the scan are much more detailed than standard X-rays.

Magnetic Resonance Imaging (MRI) Scan

The *magnetic resonance imagining (MRI) scan* is another type of scan that you may undergo. The scanning machine uses a combination of powerful magnets, radio

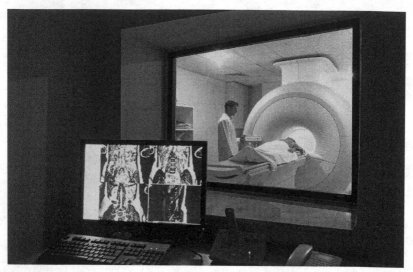

A magnetic resonance imaging (MRI) scan can detect abnormal tissue in the colon and can determine whether cancer has spread. The scan uses a large magnet, radio waves, and a computer to produce pictures; later, physicians view the scan results on a computer screen, as shown in the lower left corner.

frequency, and computers to take pictures of your soft tissues, bones, and other internal body structures. In some situations, an MRI is more effective in detecting abnormal tissues than other scans are. The MRI can also help determine whether a cancer has spread outside the colon or rectum.

For this test, you lie on an examination table that slides into a large, hollow tube. Because the MRI uses a powerful magnetic field, you cannot wear jewelry during the scan. Nor should you have any other metals with you, such as pens, watches, or eyeglasses, while undergoing the scan. People who should not have an MRI are those with metal screws, pins, or plates in their bodies; those with pacemakers; and those with cochlear ear implants. Also, if you are claustrophobic, talk to your doctor about taking a mild sedative prior to the test since you will spend fifteen to forty-five minutes inside the large cylinder. However, many testing centers now have "open MRIs," which you pass through without being confined to a cylinder.

Positron Emission Tomography (PET) Scan

The *positron emission tomography (PET) scan* provides internal photos that tell doctors how well organs and tissues are functioning; it allows them to observe such things as blood flow, oxygen use, and how the body uses glucose (sugar). This test is not typically used as an initial diagnostic tool, and when it is used, it's usually used in combination with a CT scan. Doctors will often use a PET scan to help stage a cancer after surgery, when you're preparing for additional treatment such as chemotherapy.

For this test, you'll be injected with a chemical that will move through your body; then, about an hour later, you'll lie on a table that will move through the scanner.

Ultrasound Test

Another diagnostic tool, an *ultrasound test* uses sound waves to produce pictures of internal organs. Ultrasound is often used to examine abdominal organs, specifically the liver, to check for any spread of colorectal cancer. The technician performing the test runs a device called a *transducer,* which resembles a microphone, over the body, and sound waves produce images on a video screen.

Transrectal ultrasound involves placing a thin probe inside the rectum. If a tumor is present, the sound waves penetrate the tumor and provide information about how deeply the cancer has invaded the rectal wall or whether it has spread to lymph nodes. This information is important for surgical treatment.

X-rays

A standard X-ray is not used to diagnose colorectal cancer; however, it provides a physician with other information. For example, a chest X-ray can be used to check for any underlying lung disease or whether a cancer has spread to the lungs. A chest X-ray is usually ordered before surgery once a colorectal cancer is diagnosed. An X-ray of the abdomen can also determine whether a tumor might be blocking the intestines. X-rays can also be done to evaluate whether a newly diagnosed cancer has spread to the bones.

After the Diagnostic Tests

After your diagnostic tests, your physician will discuss the results with you. If you are diagnosed with colorectal cancer, you will be referred to other physicians who specialize in the treatment of cancer. Before treatment, however, the cancer will be staged, to estimate the extent to which it has penetrated tissues. Then, a treatment plan will be determined based on the stage of the cancer.

Coping Emotionally

As mentioned earlier, fear and anxiety are common reactions to the diagnosis of colorectal cancer. It's important to recognize and cope with such negative emotions because they can affect your health. Anxiety and stress can lead to lack of sleep, poor appetite, weight loss, and poor judgment. Research has shown that stress caused by negative emotions can depress the immune system and may impair recovery.

Getting emotional support from family and friends will help you cope. If you have loved ones who are not nearby, you can stay in touch with them through several online sites. These websites allow you to create private pages where you can post updates about your hospital stays and treatments without making multiple phone calls or sending e-mails. You may also wish to consider contacting psychologists, counselors, ministers, or chaplains. Having good emotional support plays an important role in your journey through diagnosis and treatment.

Finding Support Services

Your health care team will likely have suggestions for you on where to find services for you and your family. Also, you can call the National Cancer Institute. *See* the Resources section at the back of the book.

Information specialists there will help you locate programs, services, and publications. You can speak with a specialist by calling 1-800-4-CANCER. Or, you can interact with a specialist online by going to "Live Help" at www.cancer.gov.

3   STAGING COLORECTAL CANCER

The process of *staging* a newly discovered colorectal cancer involves determining the stage of the cancer's growth. For example, is the cancer at an early stage, meaning it has not spread beyond the colon or rectum? Or, has the cancer spread outside the colorectal wall, in which case it would be considered to be at a more advanced stage. Knowing the stage of a cancer is important because it helps doctors determine the treatment plan to follow.

There are two types of staging—clinical and pathological. The clinical stage is based on your doctor's clinical findings—diagnostic tests, including X-rays, scans, and biopsies—prior to any treatment. The pathological stage is based on clinical findings along with analysis of tissue and tumor samples after surgery, a common treatment for colorectal cancer. The staging based on the pathology report is the more accurate of the two types of staging, since tissue samples taken at the time of surgery may provide more-specific information about any spread of the cancer.

How Cancer Spreads

There are three ways cancer spreads. It can spread through surrounding tissue, through the lymph system, or through blood. It can spread through surrounding tissue by first growing through the inner lining of the colon into

Areas to Which Colorectal Cancer Can Spread

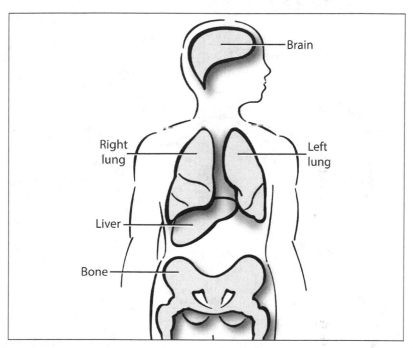

Colorectal cancer most often spreads to the liver, but it can also spread to other parts of the body, including bones, brain, lining of the abdominal cavity, lungs, or to distant lymph nodes.

the middle layer and ultimately through the outermost layer.

If the cancer extends through the entire colon wall, it can invade the adjacent *lymph nodes*. The lymph nodes are glands that filter the blood for infectious organisms as part of your immune system. There are hundreds of lymph nodes throughout your body. They are normally the size of a raisin when not inflamed or affected by cancer. You may notice that when you have a sore throat, the lymph nodes in your neck become enlarged because of the infection. In people with colorectal cancer, the lymph nodes adjacent to the tumor can be invaded by cancer cells.

Once cancer cells get into the lymph nodes, tumor cells can escape into the bloodstream and travel throughout the body. Beyond the lymph nodes, the liver is the most common site for cancer to spread. This occurs because the blood supply from the entire colon drains into the liver first. Any tumor cells in the blood leaving the colon will first become lodged in the liver.

Colorectal cancer may also spread to the brain, bones, lining of the abdominal organs, lungs, or distant lymph nodes.

Before your doctor can fully stage your colorectal cancer, he or she needs to answer the following questions:

- What is the extent of tumor growth through the colon wall?

- Are the lymph nodes near the cancer involved with the tumor?

- Has the cancer spread to other organs?

The answers to the first two questions can only be obtained after you undergo surgery and the cancerous tissue and lymph nodes are removed.

Pathology Report

After surgery, a *pathologist*, a doctor who examines tissues and organs for diseases, will perform laboratory tests on the tissue removed. Once testing of the tissue specimens is complete, he or she will deliver a written pathology report. This report will tell your physician whether the cancer has spread through the colorectal wall and whether lymph nodes are involved. It usually takes two to four days after surgery to obtain a final pathology report. The pathology report will determine your cancer stage, taking into consideration the factors listed below.

Type of Cancer Cells Present

Once the abnormal tissue is studied by the pathologist, the type of cancer cells present can be determined.

32

The types include benign, precancerous, noninvasive, and invasive. As mentioned earlier, *benign* means noncancerous. *Precancerous* means the growth has the potential to become cancer. *Noninvasive* means the cancer is limited to the lining of the colon. *Invasive* cancers are those that have invaded into or beyond the wall of the colon.

Degree of Differentiation

The degree of differentiation refers to how much the cancer cells resemble the normal cells. There are three degrees of differentiation: poorly, moderately, and well-differentiated. Poorly differentiated cancer cells are chaotic, more aggressive than the other two types, and have the worst prognosis. Well-differentiated cancer cells are not as aggressive and and have the best prognosis.

Spread to Blood Vessels

Known as *extramural venous invasion*, this condition means the cancer cells have invaded the walls of the small blood vessels surrounding the tumor and have the potential to leak into the bloodstream. This is not a favorable characteristic, as it increases the risk of spread to other organs in the body.

Resection Margins

The term *resection* refers to the surgical removal of a cancer. The *resection margins* refer to the tissue in the margins, or around the edges, of the tumor. The pathologist will analyze these tissues for evidence of cancer cells. If the resection margins are free of cancer cells, it's an indication that all the cancerous tissue was removed during the surgery. But if the resection margins contain cancer cells, further treatment will be required.

Extent of Tumor Growth

This part of the report describes how far the cancer has grown into the colorectal wall. The best-case scenario has the tumor confined to the inner layer. The worst-case scenario has the tumor growing through all the layers and invading the *pericolonic fat.* In such a case, the chances are high for *recurrence* of the cancer. In addition, the farther a cancer grows through the colorectal wall, the greater the chance of it spreading to the lymph nodes.

Lymph Node Involvement

The report will tell whether cancer has invaded any lymph nodes. If the lymph nodes are negative, it means no cancerous cells were found in the lymph nodes. According to today's standard of care, if at least twelve lymph nodes are negative, the surgery is considered successful in removing all the cancer.

A report of positive lymph nodes means cancer cells are present and further treatment will be needed. In addition, the number of lymph nodes involved is a factor in determining prognosis.

Stages of Colon Cancer

Taking all the information from the pathology report, doctors will classify the stage of your cancer. The stages range from 0 to IV.

Stage 0: In stage 0, abnormal cells are found in the innermost lining of the colon. These abnormal cells may become cancer and spread into nearby normal tissue. This stage is also called carcinoma *in situ.*

Stage I: Cancer has formed and spread beyond the innermost tissue layer of the colon wall to the middle layers.

Stage II: In stage II, colon cancer is divided into stages IIA and IIB.

Stage IIA: Cancer has spread beyond the middle tissue layers of the colon wall or has spread to nearby tissues around the colon or rectum.

Stages of Rectal Cancer

Stage I

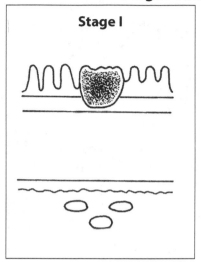

Stage I: The cancer has not spread to the colon wall.

Stage II

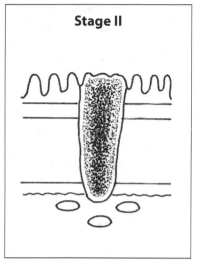

Stage II: The cancer has spread to the middle layers of the colon wall.

Stage III

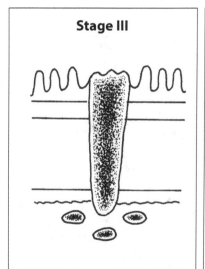

Stage III: the cancer has spread to nearby tissues and lymph nodes.

Stage IV

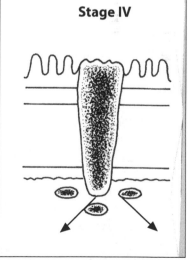

Stage IV: the cancer has spread to other organs such as the liver and lung.

Stage IIB: Cancer has spread beyond the colon wall into nearby organs and/or through the *peritoneum*.

Stage III: In stage III, colon cancer is divided into stage IIIA, stage IIIB, and stage IIIC.

Stage IIIA: Cancer has spread from the innermost tissue layer of the colon wall to the middle layers and has spread to as many as three lymph nodes.

Stage IIIB: Cancer has spread to as many as three nearby lymph nodes and has spread beyond the middle tissue layers of the colon wall, or to nearby tissues around the colon or rectum, or beyond the colon wall into nearby organs and/or through the peritoneum.

Stage IIIC: Cancer has spread to four or more nearby lymph nodes and has spread to or beyond the middle tissue layers of the colon wall, or to nearby tissues around the colon or rectum, or to nearby organs and/or through the peritoneum.

Stage IV: Cancer may have spread to nearby lymph nodes and has spread to other parts of the body, such as the liver or lungs.

Stages of Rectal Cancer

Stage 0: In stage 0, abnormal cells are found in the innermost lining of the rectum. These abnormal cells may become cancer and spread into nearby normal tissue. Stage 0 is also called carcinoma *in situ*.

Stage I: In stage I, cancer has formed and spread beyond the innermost lining of the rectum to the second and third layers and involves the inside wall of the rectum, but it has not spread to the outer wall of the rectum or outside the rectum.

Stage II: In stage II, cancer has spread outside the rectum to nearby tissue, but it has not gone into the lymph nodes.

Stage III: In stage III, cancer has spread to nearby lymph nodes, but it has not spread to other parts of the body.

Stage IV: In stage IV, cancer has spread to other parts of the body, such as the liver, lungs, or ovaries.

Note: If you wish to learn more-specific information about the system doctors use for classifying the extent to which a cancer has spread, see the "TNM Classification System" in the Appendix.

Treatment Planning

As soon as the stage of a cancer is determined, doctors can recommend the best type of treatment. For an early-stage colon or rectal cancer, treatment may involve surgery alone; in some cases chemotherapy or radiation may also be recommended. For other stages of colon or rectal cancer, most treatment plans involve surgery along with chemotherapy or radiation or a combination of both chemotherapy and radiation.

In the chapters that follow, you'll read about each of these treatment options.

4 SURGERY

If colorectal cancer has not spread to other organs, surgery is the primary treatment and offers the best chance for a cure. The goal of any operation for colorectal cancer is to remove the portion of the colon or rectum that contains the growing cancer, along with the surrounding lymph nodes.

Colorectal surgery is performed by general surgeons and colorectal surgeons. These physicians may perform one of several different types of surgery, depending on the location and stage of your cancer.

Approaches to Colon and Rectal Surgery

There are three basic approaches to surgery for colon and rectal cancer. The type your surgeon recommends will depend on factors such as where your cancer is growing and how deeply it has spread.

Open Surgery

The traditional approach to colon and rectal surgery is called an *open surgery*. The term *open* refers to the surgeon opening the abdomen to perform the surgery. A twelve-inch incision is made in the mid abdomen. Approximately 50 percent of colon and rectal surgeries are performed with this approach, making it the most commonly used.

Laparoscopic Surgery

Also called *minimally invasive surgery*, the *laparo-scopic* approach requires smaller incisions, which means less pain after surgery, quicker recovery, and less scaring. For these procedures, three incisions, approximately one inch in length, are made in the abdomen along with one six-inch incision. Then, a thin, fiber-optic camera is inserted into the abdomen. This camera sends pictures to several television monitors, essentially becoming the "eyes" of the surgeons as they manipulate small, hand-held instruments during the operation. The surgeon performs the operation while standing by the patient. Approximately 45 percent of colon and rectal surgeries are performed with this approach.

Robotic Surgery

As the name implies, for this surgery a surgeon uses robotic arms to perform the surgery. Three one-inch incisions are made along with a six- to twelve-inch incision. Surgeons view the colon on television monitors as they perform the surgery with robotic arms. Rather than standing next to the operating table, the surgeon controls the robotic arms while seated at a console in the operating room. These robotic operations are more complex for surgeons to perform, compared to traditional open surgery; only about 5 percent of colon and rectal surgeries are performed robotically; however, such robotic surgery is available in most cities and at many community hospitals.

Surgeries for Colon Cancer

Polyp Removal

The surgery to remove a polyp is called a *polyp-ectomy*. The procedure is performed by a surgeon or a gastroenterologist, a physician who treats diseases of the gastrointestinal tract and liver. Polyp removal is often done during a colonoscopy. The doctor uses an assort-

Surgeries for Colorectal Cancer

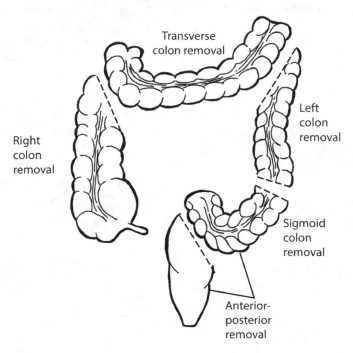

Transverse colon removal

Left colon removal

Right colon removal

Sigmoid colon removal

Anterior-posterior removal

ment of wires, snares, and small forceps to remove a polyp through the colonoscope while you are sedated. The procedure is usually done on an outpatient basis.

Most polyps that are under one inch in diameter and growing on a stalk, like a mushroom, can be removed this way. However, polyps larger than one inch in diameter, broad based, or containing cancer cells require an operation to remove a part of the colon and the surrounding lymph nodes.

Partial Removal of the Colon

The most common type of surgery for colon cancer is removal of part of the colon. This is called a *partial colectomy*. This operation may be performed with either of open, laparoscopic, or robotic techniques. The term *open* refers to the fact that an incision is made in the

Incisions for Colon Surgery

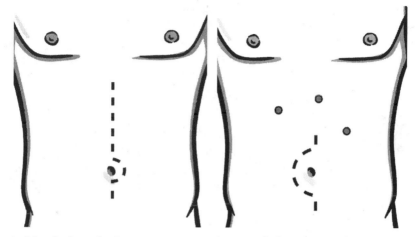

Incision for "open" colon surgery.   Incisions for laproscopic colon surgery.

abdomen to "open" it. In this case, a twelve-inch incision is made in the mid abdomen. During the operation,
the surgeon removes the segment of the colon that is
cancerous. This is major surgery and requires general
anesthesia.

The type of operation needed depends on where the
tumor is located. If the cancer is located in the right colon,
the operation is called a *right colectomy* since only the
right part of the colon is removed. To remove a cancer
in the transverse colon, a *transverse colectomy* is needed.
The transverse colon is the middle part of the large intestine that passes across the abdomen from right to left
below the stomach. A cancer located in the left colon is
removed by a *left colectomy*. One located in the sigmoid
colon is removed by a *sigmoid colectomy*. This part of the
colon is the S-shaped part of the large intestine, leading
into the rectum.

When performing a partial colectomy, a surgeon
removes approximately six inches of healthy colon on
both ends of the cancerous segment. The six inches of

Robotic Surgery Incision

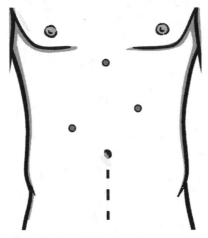

To perform robotic surgery, a surgeon makes three small incisions and one longer one in the lower abdomen.

normal colon tissue is referred to as the "margins" of the colon after the surgical procedure. An adequate margin of normal colon tissue minimizes the risk of the cancer coming back in the same area after the two ends are reconnected.

A surgeon also removes lymph nodes in the fatty tissue next to the cancerous segment; the lymph nodes are used to help determine the stage of the cancer.

After the cancerous section of the colon is removed, the surgeon reattaches the two ends of the colon. They are joined together by either sutures or metal staples. If sutures are used, your body will absorb them over several months. If metal staples are used, they are left in place permanently. Both techniques are equally effective.

The surgery takes from one to three hours and commonly involves a three- to seven-day stay in the hospital.

Removal of All or Most of the Colon

A surgical procedure to remove more than 90 percent of the colon is called a *subtotal colectomy*. It's not a common operation; however, it may be necessary when a person has two separate colon cancers in two different parts of the colon. During this major operation, the surgeon is still able to reattach both ends of normal colon after the two cancerous segments are removed.

A *total colectomy* removes the entire colon. Again, this is not a common operation for colon cancer. It is generally performed for other diseases of the colon.

This operation may be performed with either of the minimally invasive techniques; or it may be done with the open approach. Both of these operations take about three hours and involve a seven-day recovery in the hospital.

Surgeries for Rectal Cancer

Surgery for rectal cancer may be a simple procedure, such as the removal of a polyp in the rectum, or to a more extensive operation such as removal of part or all of the rectum, or anus.

Polyp Removal

Most polyps in the rectum can also be removed at the time of a colonoscopy. However, rectal polyps with a broad base and greater than one inch in diameter may be difficult to remove without an operation. In addition, polyps found to have cancer in them once removed by the colonoscope may require more-extensive surgery.

Removal of Cancerous Tissue through the Anus

In some cases, a polyp or early cancer in the rectum can be surgically removed through the anus. This is a unique approach because it does not involve a large incision through the middle of the abdomen. By operating through the anus, there is less trauma to the body

43

and less physical pain. This surgical approach is called a *transanal excision.*

After this operation, radiation treatment may be needed to kill any cancer cells left behind. The operation is carried out under general anesthesia and takes about one hour. It can be performed in an outpatient setting or in a hospital. Some patients may need to stay overnight in the hospital.

Removal of Lower Colon and Upper Section of the Rectum

This operation removes a cancer located in the lower one-third of the sigmoid colon or upper two-thirds of the rectum. It is called a *low anterior resection.* This is a major operation, in which the surgeon removes a twelve-inch portion of the lower colon and upper rectum. Adjacent lymph nodes are also removed. After removing the cancerous segment, the surgeon reattaches the two free ends together so normal bowel movements can occur.

This operation may be performed laparoscopically, robotically, or an open approach may be used. The hospital stay is typically at least seven days.

Surgical Removal of the Rectum

Rectal cancer is the most common reason for the removal of the rectum. The last six inches of your large intestine is made up of your rectum and anal area. When a cancer is located within six inches of the outside of the anus, an operation to remove the rectum may offer the best chance of a cure. Called a *proctectomy,* this procedure removes part of all or the rectum.

This operation involves a twelve-inch vertical incision in your abdomen; the surgery takes three hours and requires general anesthesia. The medical term for this procedure is *open anterior-posterior resection.* As mentioned earlier, a resection refers to surgical removal of tissue or structure.

What Is an Ostomy?

When the anus is removed, it is no longer possible to have normal bowel movements. Instead, an artificially created hole is made in the abdomen so that waste can flow out of the body and into a bag that is worn externally. Such a bag is called an *ostomy;* if the ostomy is connected to the colon, the bag is called a *colostomy.* When a piece of the small intestine is used to create an ostomy, it's called an *ileostomy.*

In some cases, if a rectal cancer is large, it can be shrunk with chemotherapy and radiation before surgery.

By shrinking the tumor, the operation can be completed by the surgeon's attaching the end of the colon to the anus; this eliminates the need for a colostomy bag.

However, in some cases, the surgeon must remove both the rectum and anus. Removal of both will require a colostomy. To create the colostomy, the surgeons connect the colon to an opening on the surface of the lower abdomen. An external colostomy bag is attached to the new opening; fecal matter will no longer pass through the anus, but will pass into this bag. You'll learn more about colostomies at the end of this chapter.

Finding an Experienced Surgeon

In addition to discussing whether you'll have an open surgery or a minimally invasive procedure (laparoscopic or robotic), you'll want to be sure your surgeon is experienced. Having an experienced surgeon perform your surgery will minimize your risk of complications and give you the best chance for a good outcome. General surgeons and colorectal surgeons perform both traditional open and minimally invasive colorectal surgery. Ask the surgeon three questions. The first is: How many colorectal operations do you perform a year? Experienced surgeons are performing at least twenty major colorectal operations a year.

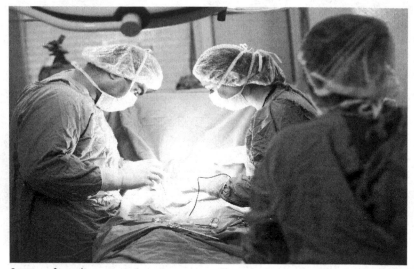

Surgery for colon cancer is major surgery. The most common procedure involves removal of a portion of the colon.

Secondly, ask a surgeon what percentage of his or her surgeries are performed laparoscopically or robotically. An experienced surgeon should be performing at least 50 percent of surgeries with these two minimally invasive approaches.

Finally, ask the surgeon: What are the two main complications of my operation and how often do they occur in your patients every year? The responses should be surgical site infections, which occur at a rate of 15 to 20 percent, and leaking problems where two ends of colon are reconnected after surgery. (Bowel leakage can occur.) An acceptable complication rate for this leakage is 5 to 10 percent of patients.

Preparation for Colon or Rectal Surgery

Prior to any colorectal operation, your surgeon will prescribed a *bowel prep* to clean your colon. This will involve drinking a solution to flush your colon. You will also be asked to stay on a liquid diet for one or two days prior to your operation.

Undergoing Surgery

After you arrive at the hospital on the morning of your surgery, you will be admitted and escorted to a room, where you'll change into a hospital gown. A nurse will place an intravenous (IV) line in a vein in your arm and an anesthesiologist, who will administer your anesthesia, and his or her assistant will visit you prior to surgery. The anesthesiologist will ask you questions about such things as your past experience with surgery and anesthesia, whether you have any drug allergies, and whether you have any chronic medical problems.

After you are in the operating room, the anesthesiologist and the assistant will administer the anesthesia into your IV, and they will monitor you during the operation.

After you receive the anesthesia, you will fall asleep within seconds. You won't be able to feel or hear anything. Then, a nasogastric tube will be placed down your throat and into your stomach; this tube will suction out any accumulation of fluid that could cause vomiting. A catheter will also be placed in your bladder while you are asleep to monitor your urine output during the surgery. This catheter will likely be left in overnight and removed within twenty-four to forty-eight hours after your operation. Compression devices will also be placed on your legs to reduce the risk of blood clots forming; these devices use cuffs around the legs that fill with air and squeeze your legs.

During the operation, your surgeon will remove the cancerous segment of your colon and reconnect the two free ends together. Your surgeon will also visually inspect all the other organs in your abdominal cavity to look for evidence that the cancer has spread. If a suspicious nodule or mass is found, especially in the liver, the surgeon will remove a piece of tissue for laboratory examination (biopsy).

After the operation is complete, the nasogastric tube is removed before you wake up; however, the surgeon may leave the nasogastric tube in place so it can continue to suction any fluid buildup over the next two to four days. Once the anesthesiologist gives the okay, you will be taken to the recovery room.

In the recovery room, your vital signs (blood pressure, heart rate, and respiration rate) will be closely monitored and checked by the nurses. When your anesthesiologist determines that you are stable, you'll be moved to a hospital room.

Recovery in the Hospital

Barring any major complications, you will need five to seven days in the hospital to recover from traditional, open surgery for colorectal cancer surgery. If you have had a minimally invasive surgery, you may need to stay less time—three to four days.

While you are in the hospital, your surgeon, or a member of his or her team, will monitor your progress. The surgeon will determine: when to remove tubes or catheters, when to decrease your pain medicine, when to have your dressing changed, when you should get out of bed, and when to advance your diet. All these decisions are influenced by how soon your bodily functions return to normal; the physical stress from the operation typically interrupts body functions, and it may take a few days for these functions to return to normal.

Pain Management after Surgery

Prior to surgery, be sure to discuss ways to manage your postoperative pain with your surgeon. Don't wait until you're groggy after surgery to discuss this important issue.

There are several methods for controlling pain. You can be given periodic injections of narcotic drugs. You can be hooked up to a *patient-controlled anesthesia*

48

(PCA) pump that administers a continuous dose of narcotics over a twenty-four-hour period. The PCA pump also allows you to administer additional narcotic booster injections through a handheld device if the pain worsens. The PCA pump provides steadier, more even postoperative pain control than traditional injections.

An *epidural catheter* is another form of pain management. The catheter is a tiny, soft plastic tube that an anesthesiologist inserts in the middle of your back and guides close to your spinal cord. The medication affects the nerves that cause you to feel pain from the surgery. The catheter may be left in place for several days after surgery. It is an effective way to control pain after major abdominal operations.

Once you begin to drink liquids or eat solid food, your surgeon will likely switch from intravenous pain medications to oral medications. These should be taken as directed, to stay ahead of the pain. Don't wait until you're in pain to take the medications.

Your postoperative pain should lessen with each passing day. If your pain is not being adequately controlled, tell your nurse or your surgeon. Tolerating pain should not be part of the normal healing process. You are not being a bothersome patient by asking for help with pain relief.

Regaining Bowel Function

It is normal for your bowel function to be interrupted after colorectal surgery. You will need to regain normal bowel function and tolerate a regular diet before being released from the hospital. Several factors affect the return of normal bowel function. First, muscle or nerve problems may temporarily disrupt the normal coordinated muscle contractions of the intestines, slowing or stopping the movement of food and fluid through the digestive system. Narcotic pain medications will also slow your intestines. Inactivity after your operation will also contribute to the slowing of your intestine.

This is why walking twenty-four hours after your operation is encouraged. Chewing gum after your operation has been shown to speed up your bowel function after surgery. Your surgeon may also prescribe a medication, *Entereg,* to be taken immediately before your operation and for several days after; this medication will lessen the time it takes to return to normal bowel function.

Keeping the Lungs Expanded

After your operation, the nurses caring for you will tell you to practice deep breathing and coughing. Placing a pillow on your stomach and holding it as you cough will also ease the pain immediately after surgery. Deep breaths help keep the lungs expanded to prevent pneumonia. If you smoke or have a history of lung disease, deep breathing is especially important.

Because deep breathing hurts after major abdominal surgery, it is natural to want to take short, incomplete breaths. Concentrate on your breathing while recovering in the hospital. An *incentive spirometer* can help you keep your lungs expanded. This is a tubelike device you breathe through that has a gauge that shows how well your lungs expand by measuring how deep your breathing is.

Blood Tests

For several days after your operation, blood will be taken from your arm each morning to evaluate your blood count. Since these lab values will fluctuate after major abdominal surgery, your surgeon needs to monitor them during recovery.

If your blood count drops too low, you may require a transfusion. A low blood count can lead to low blood pressure, fatigue, and potentially a heart attack if you

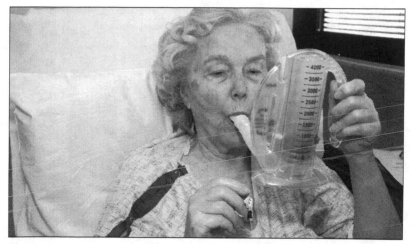

Blowing into an incentive spirometer helps keep the lungs expanded after surgery. *Photo by CMSP*

have a history of heart problems. Other abnormalities in the blood can lead to abnormal heart rhythms and seizures and can prolong the inactivity of the intestines following surgery.

Regaining Mobility

Getting out of bed and walking in your room or in the hallway as soon as you are physically able is also important for a fast, uncomplicated recovery. Walking gets the blood circulating, prevents blood clots from forming, and may help you regain intestinal function more quickly. Walking, like coughing and deep breathing, will cause some initial discomfort. However, as each day passes, it will become easier. Walking may be difficult while you're connected to tubes and intravenous lines. The nurses or a therapist will assist you.

Planning for Additional Treatment

Before you leave the hospital or shortly thereafter, your surgeon will talk to you about your pathology report. The pathology report describes the stage of your cancer and whether or not you need further treatment. Today, many patients are undergoing minimally invasive colorectal surgery and leaving the hospital before their pathology report has been completed. If additional treatment is needed, your surgeon will call in a medical oncologist for consultation. A *medical oncologist* is a doctor who treats cancer.

Discharge from the Hospital

As your hospital stay draws to an end, you should be walking as much as possible and eating normal food. Your bowel movements should be close to normal, and the pain from your incision should be adequately controlled with oral pain medication.

On the day you're discharged from the hospital, you will be given instructions for managing postoperative pain; usually, you will be given a prescription for painkillers. You'll also be given guidelines for levels of activity that are appropriate for you, along with instructions for such activities as bathing.

If your surgeon used metal staples to close your incision, they will need to be removed during a follow-up office appointment, usually in seven to ten days. (These staples are different from those used internally to connect the segments of your colon.)

Possible Complications of Colorectal Surgery

The risk for complications after colorectal cancer surgery depends on a number of factors. Your overall health and any preexisting medical conditions can affect whether you develop complications. You have a slightly higher risk for developing complications if you have high blood pressure, lung disease, or diabetes, or if you are obese or if you are a smoker. In these cases, a common complication is infections at the incision site. Your risk for complications is minimal if you are healthy, do not smoke, and are physically active.

Whether your surgery is planned or performed on an emergency basis also impacts your risk for complications. A planned operation takes place in a controlled setting under optimum conditions so the risks are small. Emergency surgery has a higher complication rate.

Complications following colorectal surgery are relatively rare, occurring in less than 5 percent of patients. However, the complications can be life threatening if they aren't recognized and treated immediately. Possible complications include heart attack, pneumonia, wound infection, blood clots in the legs (with potential spread to the lungs), or an intra-abdominal infection or associated abscess due to a leak in the colon. Another complication, called a *fistula* is an abnormal connection between the intestine and the skin. A fistula occurs when the intestine is punctured and stool leaks out. It can lead to a serious infection requiring antibiotics. Most fistulas, however, heal spontaneously and do not require surgery.

Even in the 5 percent of patients who do experience postsurgical complications, most respond to treatment and do not require further surgery.

Recovery at Home

Recovering at home after colorectal cancer surgery can take four to eight weeks. While at home, it is normal to initially not have much of an appetite. Most people lose ten to twenty pounds following surgery. Your appetite will improve over the next several weeks. Most often, you'll be free to eat whatever you'd like.

Watch for any signs of infection—fever, any drainage, redness, increasing pain from your abdominal incision, and coughing up dark sputum. All these are warning signs of infection, and your surgeon needs to be notified immediately. Your bowel habits should quickly return to normal once you return home. Persistent diarrhea while at home is not normal. Let your surgeon know if this occurs. Persistent nausea, abdominal pain, and vomiting are also not normal and also should be reported.

Do not expect to have a normal energy level right away. It may take one to two months for your energy to return to the preoperative level. Do not try to do too much too fast. Limit your activities, and do not expect to return to work for at least one month. Expect your energy level to fluctuate, alternating between good days and bad days. This is completely normal after major colorectal surgery.

In addition to being a physical strain, recovering at home from colorectal cancer surgery can be full of emotional ups and downs. This kind of mental stress is especially prevalent when you are at home, inactive, and recovering, with plenty of time to think. Try to keep busy at home with hobbies and things that exercise your mental capabilities.

Do not be afraid to open up to family and friends. Talk with them about how you're feeling, your fears, and your concerns. Try to maintain a positive outlook. Some people find comfort in cancer support groups; such groups can provide moral support and practical advice for recovery. Also, consider talking with friends, neighbors, and coworkers who have had cancer and have gone through treatment.

If You Need a Colostomy

As mentioned earlier, colostomy refers to the creation of an opening in the lower abdomen. A colostomy bag, attached to the opening, collects waste. According to the National Cancer Institute, about 15 percent of people who undergo surgery for colorectal cancer require a permanent colostomy. Whether you need a colostomy depends upon several factors. The size and location of your tumor is a consideration. Also, is your surgery scheduled or is it performed on an emergency basis? When a surgeon performs an operation in an

Colostomy Bag

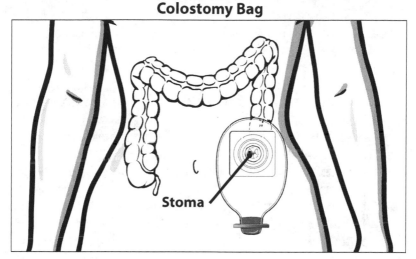

Stoma

When it's necessary for the surgeon to remove the anus, an external colostomy bag is needed to collect waste. About 15 percent of people with colorectal cancer require a colostomy.

emergency, such as when a colon cancer is obstructing the intestines, there is no time to clean the colon out. When the colon is not cleansed, the risk of infection markedly increases. An infection may create the need for a colostomy.

Temporary Colostomy

Sometimes, a *temporary colostomy* is required after emergency colon surgery. In these cases, a colostomy helps avoid serious infections. For example, you may need emergency surgery to have a blockage in your colon removed. Or, you may need emergency surgery if cancer has perforated the colon wall, causing feces and bacteria to spill into the abdomen. Since there is no time to cleanse the colon prior to surgery, the risk of infection is high if two ends of a "dirty" colon are sewn together after a cancerous segment has been removed. The best way to minimize this risk is to perform a temporary colostomy at the time of the operation.

A temporary colostomy usually remains in place for four to six months, enough time for healing after the surgery. Then, in another operation, the surgeon can go back and reconnect the colon sections. This reversal of the colostomy is called a *colostomy takedown*. It is a major operation that takes several hours and involves general anesthesia and a week's recovery in the hospital. Colostomy takedown restores normal bowel function.

A temporary *ileostomy* is sometimes performed during major colorectal surgery. This procedure protects the colon connection. An ileostomy involves creating an opening to the skin with a segment of small intestine. The opening is usually placed on the right side of your body. A temporary ileostomy can be reversed to re-create normal bowel function in four to six weeks after surgery.

Permanent Colostomy

A *permanent colostomy* is required if the cancer is located in the rectum close to the anus and the surgeon must remove the entire rectum and part of the colon. In this case, it is no longer possible to reattach the colon to the rectum. As a result, a colostomy is needed.

If you have a colostomy, its location on your abdomen will usually be determined before surgery. For most individuals, the colostomy is located below and to the left of the navel. It is uncommon to find colostomies located elsewhere in the abdomen.

Wearing a Colostomy Bag

To attach the colostomy bag, first a plastic adhesive barrier, shaped like a doughnut, is placed around the opening in the abdomen. This opening is called a *stoma*. Then, the external plastic pouch is attached to the adhesive barrier. The pouch fits under your clothes and is usually not noticeable to others.

Colostomy Care

While you're in the hospital, you may see an *enterostomal nurse*, a registered nurse specially trained in the care of colostomies. In addition to explaining how to care for your colostomy, this nurse will provide other information such as where to get supplies in your community.

Caring for your colostomy at home is not difficult. The pouch needs to be emptied into the toilet periodically during the day as it fills up. You can empty the pouch by opening a plastic clip at its base and allowing the fecal material to spill into the toilet. After the pouch has been emptied, the plastic clip can be reattached and the bottom of the pouch closed. Most people become very adept at emptying the pouch and do not have problems with soiled garments or lingering odors. Drops of deodorizer can be dropped into the bag immediately after it is emptied. There are several specialized liquid deodorizers that may be purchased at medical supply stores.

Irrigating your colostomy with a simple saline solution will be helpful if it becomes clogged. Essentially, colostomy irrigation works like an enema. Ask your nurse or doctor about irrigation and how to do it. The plastic pouch itself usually needs to be replaced every five to seven days. The colostomy opening may be washed with soap and water.

Most people with colostomies keep extra supplies nearby just in case they are needed unexpectedly. Make sure you have plenty of supplies at home. Colostomy supplies can be obtained in some drugstores and in many medical supply stores.

You do *not* need to be on a special diet with a colostomy. However, certain foods can affect the consistency of your colostomy output. Some foods may cause diarrhea or excess gas. Other foods may cause constipation.

You can exert some control over your colostomy bowel habits by modifying your diet. By watching what you eat and eating at regular intervals, you can control when your colostomy works during the day. Ask your doctor about how foods affect your colostomy; your doctor may help you with this or may refer you to a dietician.

Emotional Support

At first, accepting the fact that you have a colostomy may be emotionally difficult. You may experience feelings of depression, frustration, anger, sadness, and isolation. You may withdraw from family and friends. It's important to realize that all these feelings and reactions are common. Talk with those you trust—your physician, family members, and friends. Consider seeking out cancer and colostomy support groups in your area. They can provide valuable insights and help you cope with your new situation.

Colostomy's Effect on Sexual Activity

Many people wonder if a colostomy will affect their sex lives. Usually, individuals who have colostomies can have active sex lives. Women normally have no loss of sexual function due to a colostomy. However, some men who have had colostomies do not ejaculate, or they may have a retrograde emission, in which semen is forced backward into the bladder. This may occur because tiny nerves located deep in the pelvis, near the rectum, may be damaged during surgery. Surgeons try to avoid damaging these nerves, but if damage occurs, the emission of semen may be affected. A man's ability to attain an erection is not changed, but pleasurable sensations during sexual activity may be slightly diminished. Still, with a few changes, most individuals adapt and continue having a normal sex life.

Potential Complications

Most people do not have complications with their colostomy. However, one of the most common problems that occurs is the development of a hernia around the stoma. Symptoms of a hernia include a bulge in the skin around the stoma, problems with irrigating, or blockages. Seek medical attention if you experience any of the following symptoms:

- Severe cramps that last for more than two to three hours
- Watery discharge from the stoma for more than six hours
- No output from the colostomy for several days
- Unusual odor that lasts more than a week
- Bleeding from the stoma or seeing blood in the pouch
- Stoma pulling inward or narrowing
- Chronic skin irritation

Another possible problem is rubbing or irritation from the pouch that may cause skin abrasions; your physician may prescribe topical ointments.

Life after Receiving a Colostomy

People with colostomies live normal, active lives. A colostomy does not mean your lifestyle needs to change dramatically. Initially, a colostomy presents physical and emotional challenges. However, with the proper education and support, these challenges can be overcome. After you've recovered from your operation, you can exercise, wear normal clothes, and return to work without feeling awkward or embarrassed.

5 CHEMOTHERAPY, TARGETED THERAPY, AND IMMUNOTHERAPY

Chemotherapy, the use of medication to attack cancer, plays a major role in cancer treatment. It is used to help cure, control, or ease the symptoms of cancer. Nearly half of all cancer patients undergo chemotherapy.

Also, your medical oncologist, who treats cancer with chemotherapy, may talk to you about targeted therapy and immunotherapy. Targeted therapies attack the inner workings of cancer cells, and immunotherapy works by strengthening the body's own immune system so it can better fight cancer.

How Chemotherapy Works

To understand how chemotherapy destroys cancer cells, it helps to know how cancer cells and normal cells grow in the body. Cancer cells reproduce quickly, and chemotherapy works by destroying quickly-growing cells.

However, there are other, normal cells in your body that also grow quickly—skin cells, hair cells, the lining of the gastrointestinal tract, and the cells in our bone marrow. Because these healthy cells also reproduce rapidly, they, too, are affected by chemotherapy; this is why one can lose hair during chemotherapy. The good news is noncancerous cells that are damaged during treatment have the ability to recover.

Chemotherapy after Surgery

In some cases, chemotherapy is given *after* surgery with the intention of killing any cancer cells that might remain after surgery. This is called *adjuvant therapy*. For colon and rectal cancer, chemotherapy is given when the cancer has spread through the wall of the colon or rectum or has entered the lymph nodes. Other factors that determine whether chemotherapy is appropriate include the type of cancer, how aggressive it is, the patient's age, and the overall health of the patient.

If you've undergone surgery, your physician will probably wait three to four weeks before beginning chemotherapy, allowing you to heal from the surgery. Most chemotherapy treatments for colon cancer after surgery continue for three to six months, with a treatment once every two weeks.

Chemotherapy before Surgery

Chemotherapy is not usually given prior to surgery. This is called *neoadjuvant therapy*. However, chemotherapy may be given in an effort to shrink a tumor. The shrinkage increases the likelihood of a surgeon being able to remove an entire tumor during surgery; the chemotherapy is also intended to kill any cancer cells that may have traveled to other parts of the body.

Chemotherapy before surgery may be recommended for rectal cancer; this is done for two reasons—to preserve the anal sphincter and to reduce the chances of cancer recurring in the rectum. When cancers are found near the anus, it is often impossible to preserve the anal sphincter with surgery alone; however, when chemotherapy is given prior to the surgery, the sphincter can be saved more than 50 percent of the time. If the sphincter is removed, the patient requires a colostomy, an opening in the abdomen for collecting waste in an external bag.

Chemotherapy before rectal cancer surgery usually lasts four to six weeks and can be given at the same time

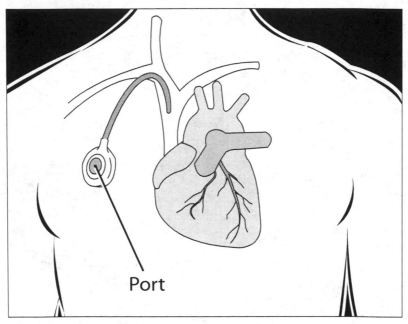

Port

Before chemotherapy begins, a surgeon may implant a port, a small reservoir, under the skin. Chemotherapy infusions will be given through this port.

as radiation. Chemotherapy can also improve outcome if given for four to six months *after* surgery. Your oncologist may talk with you about this option

Receiving Chemotherapy Treatments

Chemotherapy treatments are given in cycles— usually once every two weeks. You receive a treatment, followed by a two-week recovery period. Then, you'll have another treatment, followed by another recovery period. Why are treatments given in cycles? As explained earlier, chemotherapy kills the cancer cells that are rapidly dividing; however, it won't affect those cells that are at rest. By giving the treatments in cycles, the effort is intensified to kill cancer cells when they are in the reproduction phase. The time off between treatments also helps normal tissues recover.

Most chemotherapy treatments are given intravenously (through a needle into a vein). These treatments are called *infusions*. Treatment in pill form would seem easier, but stomach acids and enzymes break down some medications and prevent them from working effectively.

Chemotherapy infusions are given in an outpatient setting, usually in a hospital's infusion center or at another outpatient site. A nurse who specializes in giving chemotherapy treatments will connect the intravenous line that delivers the chemotherapy. Before the treatment, patients are first given antinausea medication. Nurses monitor patients carefully during infusions.

While you're receiving an infusion, you'll usually be seated in a comfortable reclining chair. A treatment may last from ninety minutes to four hours, depending on the chemotherapy agents used. During this time, you'll be able to have a snack, read, watch television, use a laptop computer, or have visitors.

Chemotherapy through a Port

Chemotherapy for colorectal cancer is given over an extended period of time. So, to make the treatment process more efficient and more comfortable for you, your doctor will want to avoid starting an intravenous (IV) line each time you have a treatment. Therefore, your chemotherapy may be delivered through a *port*.

A port is a small reservoir, about the size of a quarter, and often made of soft plastic. This port is surgically implanted in your chest just under the skin—usually under the collarbone. A soft, thin tube runs from the port into a large vein. The implantation of the port is an outpatient procedure, and it takes thirty to sixty minutes. Local anesthesia is used, and you may be given a mild sedative. After the procedure, a chest X-ray is done to check the positioning of the port and to make sure there is no kink in the tube.

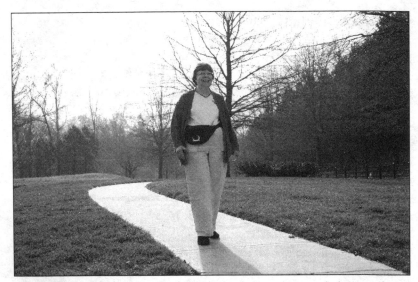

Chemotherapy treatments are often delivered through an ambulatory infusion pump, which attaches to a belt. The pump will deliver chemotherapy while you're at home. *Photo courtesy of Outpatient Infusion Systems*

From this point, the intravenous infusion line will be connected to this port. When not in use, the port is covered with a bandage; after the small incision heals, no bandage is needed. The port requires no special care by the patient; it doesn't break through the skin and shouldn't limit daily activities.

Ports rarely create complications; however, pain, redness, or swelling may indicate infection or clotting. You should report any such symptoms to your doctor immediately. Once you have completed your treatments, your port can be removed.

Chemotherapy through a Pump

When you are receiving an infusion at a treatment center, your chemotherapy drug may flow from an IV bag, which hangs from a pole. A needle that is attached to a soft, plastic tube leading from the pump is inserted into your port.

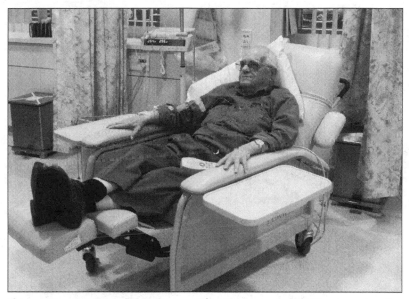

This man is receiving a chemotherapy infusion at an outpatient treatment center. Treatments are typically given in cycles—every two weeks.

After you've finished such treatment, your oncologist may want you to continue receiving the chemotherapy drug for usually forty-eight hours. You will be asked to wear an *ambulatory infusion pump,* a lightweight, battery-operated pump in a small bag that attaches to a waist belt. This pump releases the chemotherapy drug into the bloodstream at a slow, even, continuous rate. The pump is portable, and you'll wear it around the clock, even while you sleep.

Being Monitored during Treatment

You'll be monitored closely by your medical team while you're undergoing chemotherapy. You'll have routine appointments for blood testing; your doctor will be watching for such things as lowered red blood cell count, white blood cell count, or platelet count. Red blood cells carry proteins and oxygen from the lungs to the rest of the body. If these cells are reduced, it can affect energy

---

What Is KRAS Testing?

The KRAS gene is a protein that is involved in regulating cell division. Some tumors have proteins, called *epidermal growth factor receptors,* that are found on the surface of tumors; these proteins help cancer grow.

KRAS testing involves the microscopic examination of tumor tissue after surgery, helping oncologists determine which chemotherapy agents will work better for some patients and not others. People with metastatic cancer, whose tumors have what are considered normal KRAS genes, respond significantly better to certain chemotherapy agents, which inhibit cancer cells' growth. However, patients who have altered (or mutated) KRAS genes do not respond to such agents.

KRAS testing involves doing a laboratory analysis on sample tissues after surgery. About 60 percent of individuals are believed to have normal KRAS genes, which means they may respond better to specific chemotherapy agents.

---

levels as well as heart and brain function. A drop in white blood cells could put you at risk for infections, and a low platelet count could increase risk of bleeding or bruising.

In most people, blood counts drop to their lowest levels seven to ten days after each treatment. This lowest point is called the *nadir.* When you are at your nadir, your immune system is weakened, and you can be susceptible to viruses and infections. You may receive medications that boost your white blood cell count during this period. Your doctor may also choose to decrease the dose of the chemotherapy to prevent any of the blood counts from dropping too low.

Chemotherapy Medications

The medications used for chemotherapy consist of a group of different drugs, just as the term *antibiotics* refers to many different types of medications. Chemotherapy medications may be used alone, or they may be combined with other chemotherapy agents, usually no more than two to three at one time.

Some chemotherapy drugs work by attacking the cancer cells' DNA, which is a cell's "blueprint" for growing and reproducing. These drugs interrupt the cells' ability to reproduce. Some agents work by slowing down or stopping the cell division process. Other chemotherapy drugs work by attacking cell molecules, such as those involved with blood-vessel formation.

Side Effects of Chemotherapy

Chemotherapy used to treat colon and rectal cancer is generally well tolerated by most people. As mentioned earlier, chemotherapy kills cancer cells that are rapidly reproducing. However, chemotherapy drugs will also attack the normal, healthy cells that reproduce rapidly. This action causes side effects.

The type of chemotherapy you receive, the dosage, and the duration of your treatment are factors in the types of side effects that you may experience. It's important to note that not all patients experience every side effect, and when side effects do occur, they can usually be managed with oral medications you can take at home. Most side effects subside once a treatments ends. A list of potential side effects follows.

Diarrhea

One of the most common side effects of chemotherapy used to treat colorectal cancer is diarrhea. It is caused by chemotherapy acting on the lining of the stomach and intestines. Abdominal cramping can also accompany diarrhea. Both may last several hours to several days. The concern about diarrhea is that, if not treated, it can lead to dehydration. If diarrhea becomes severe, you may need to have fluids replaced intravenously, and hospitalization may be required.

Because diarrhea can cause the body to lose a large amount of water in a short period of time, you can also lose important minerals called *electrolytes*. If you're having diarrhea, these tips may help:

- Drink at least six to eight glasses of water daily.
- Avoid high-fiber, greasy, and spicy foods.
- Avoid sugary foods, especially those with processed sugars.
- Eat small amounts of solid food frequently throughout the day.
- Avoid coffee, caffeinated tea, and alcohol.

If diarrhea persists for more than twenty-four hours, contact your doctor. Do not take any over-the-counter medication for diarrhea without consulting your doctor.

Nausea and Vomiting

Nausea and vomiting are *not* common side effects of chemotherapy used to treat colorectal cancer. If you should experience these side effects, your oncologist can prescribe medications that will help. You can also take these medications to prevent nausea if it occurs often. If vomiting persists for twenty-four hours, notify your doctor. You may need to be admitted to the hospital for intravenous fluids and medication. Here are other tips for managing nausea and vomiting:

- Take antinausea medications as directed.
- Breathe deeply and slowly when you feel nauseous.
- Drink six to eight glasses of water daily.
- Eat small, frequent meals rather than three large ones.
- Eat and drink slowly. Chew foods well.
- Avoid rich, spicy, greasy foods.
- Suck on ice cubes, mints, or ginger candies (unless you have mouth sores).

Some people find that the smell of food cooking bothers them. If this occurs, plan to avoid the kitchen when food is being prepared.

Hair Loss

Chemotherapy can affect hair follicles, causing temporary hair loss. Although hair loss can occur anywhere on the body, it is mainly confined to the head. During chemotherapy, some patients wear hats to cover their heads and stay warm. Women may also choose scarves or wigs. To cope with hair loss, try these suggestions:

- Use mild shampoos.

- Use a soft hairbrush.

- Use low heat on your hair dryer or avoid hair-dryer use.

- Don't dye your hair, use brush rollers, or get a permanent.

- Have your hair cut short. A shorter style will make hair look thicker and fuller.

- Protect your scalp from the sun with a hat, scarf, or sunscreen.

- Apply cool cloths or cooled lotions to help the initial itchiness that comes with hair loss. Store a bottle of lotion in the refrigerator.

After your treatments are completed, hair grows back, although it may grow back a slightly different color or texture.

Neuropathy

Chemotherapy can cause *neuropathy,* which is damage to nerve endings. When this occurs, you may have pain, numbness, or tingling sensations in various parts of the body. The severity of these side effects depends on the amount of the chemotherapy agent you received and how quickly it was administered.

Commonly, neuropathy occurs in the hands and feet. It may interfere with activities such as buttoning a shirt, typing, writing, or playing a musical instrument. It's important to report these side effects to your oncologist right away, so he or she can adjust or suspend treatment before side effects become severe.

Neuropathy can also occur in the mouth, throat, or chest, usually when you drink chilled beverages or breathe in cold air. This may result in abnormal tongue sensations, choking sensations, or a sensation of pressure on your chest.

Neuropathy may be either acute or chronic. Acute neuropathy goes away within days of a chemotherapy treatment. However, chronic neuropathy can persist for weeks to months.

To help manage neuropathy, try these tips:

- Avoid cold drinks.

- Avoid handling cold objects.

- Inhale warm air, which may help with symptoms in the mouth and throat. If you live in a cold region try covering your mouth with a scarf before going outside.

- Continue to walk or stay as active as possible during chemotherapy treatment; movement can help prevent chronic neuropathy.

Neuropathy symptoms may be constant, or they may come and go. The chronic form may become irreversible if treatment continues, so oncologists usually reduce the dosages of the chemotherapy agent or stop the treatment. Medications are also available to alleviate neuropathy pain.

Infections

Fortunately, infection is not one of the most common side effects of chemotherapy for colorectal cancer. But, chemotherapy can damage cells in the bone marrow,

Palliative Chemotherapy

Palliative chemotherapy is given to provide relief from symptoms when a cancer is considered incurable. This chemotherapy is given with the goal of controlling the cancer as long as possible. Palliative chemotherapy may be an option when cancer has already spread to other organs, such as the liver, lungs, or bones at the time of initial diagnosis; sometimes such spread is not discovered until undergoing surgery. In such cases, chemotherapy may shrink the tumor and slow its growth.

which is important to infection-fighting white blood cells. When your white blood cell count is low, it may lead to a weakening of the immune system, a condition known as *neutropenia*. This condition makes you susceptible to infections. These can include blood infections, urinary infections, skin infections, and pneumonia.

Be alert for the signs of infection—fever of more than 100.4°F, shaking, chills, sweats, coughing up dark or bloody sputum, pain or burning with urination, and pain or redness around cuts. Infections can be effectively treated with antibiotics. To reduce your risk of infection, take these precautions:

- Wash your hands often during the day, especially after using the bathroom.
- Avoid anyone who has a cold, flu, measles, or chicken pox.
- Stay away from children who have recently received vaccinations.
- Clean cuts and scrapes right away.
- Wear gloves when gardening or cleaning up after pets or children.
- Use a soft toothbrush that won't hurt your gums.
- Clean your rectal area gently but thoroughly after each bowel movement. Notify your doctor or nurse if this area becomes irritated or if you have hemorrhoids.

If you feel an infection coming on, notify your doctor immediately.

Fatigue

Fatigue is a common side effect of chemotherapy. Fatigue can be brought on by a low red cell count or low white blood cell count. When your red blood cell count is low, tissues and organs are not receiving adequate oxygen. This condition is called *anemia*. If your red blood cell count drops too low, you may need a blood transfusion or medication that stimulates production of red blood cells.

Most patients on chemotherapy experience some degree of fatigue. For some, fatigue occurs around the time of a treatment. Others feel fatigued during the entire course of therapy. The fatigue may last even after chemotherapy has ended, and it may take weeks or months for you to recover your normal energy level. For normally active patients, the fatigue can be a source of frustration or even depression. Try to stay positive and remember that the fatigue is temporary. Here are a few tips for coping with fatigue:

- Keep a good sleep/wake schedule; avoid excessive sleeping during the day.

- Take one to two twenty-minute naps during the day if necessary; if more are needed discuss this with your doctor.

- Good nutrition is key! Eat healthful foods high in protein. If you don't feel hungry during mealtime, try a protein shake.

- Physical activity is a must—try to do something active every day as this will decrease chances of chronic fatigue. If any joint pain is preventing this, speak to your doctor as some physical therapy may be recommended

- Ask for help when you need it.

Impaired Blood Clotting

Chemotherapy can also cause a condition called *thrombocytopenia,* which means low blood platelet counts. Platelets are the cells that help blood to clot. Mild cases may produce no symptoms. However, if platelet counts drop low enough, symptoms may include easy bruising, which means bleeding has occurred in the small blood vessels under the skin. Shallow bleeding in the skin can also cause a purplish rash on the hands and feet. Other symptoms include spontaneous nosebleeds. In serious cases, internal bleeding may occur.

There are no medications for this condition, and physicians will usually delay or suspend chemotherapy treatment when blood platelet counts are low. This break in treatment gives the platelet count time to increase on its own. When counts drop dangerously low, blood platelet transfusions may be needed to avoid bleeding complications.

After the course of chemotherapy has ended, the low blood counts are treatable and reversible. Throughout your treatment, your doctor will check your blood counts with blood tests.

Mouth Sores

Chemotherapy can cause painful sores and ulcers on the lips, mouth, gums, and throat. The medical term for these mouth sores is *stomatitis* or *mucositis.* In addition to causing discomfort, mouth sores may make eating and drinking difficult, which may lead to dehydration. In some instances, these sores become infected. Fortunately, mouth sores disappear once the treatments have concluded. Ask your doctor about medication to treat these sores.

Stay hydrated by drinking plenty of water. Avoid spicy, sauce-based foods. Eat soft foods such as baby food, milk shakes, smoothies, yogurt, cooled oatmeal, and mashed vegetables until your condition improves. Also, medicines are available that can numb these sores, allowing more ease with eating. Here are additional suggestions for coping with mouth sores:

- Practice good oral hygiene—brush and floss.
- Use a soft-bristle brush to avoid irritating gum tissue.
- Avoid mouthwashes that contain a lot of salt or alcohol; baking soda mouthwashes may help.
- Avoid whitening toothpastes.
- If possible, have your teeth cleaned and any dental work completed before starting chemotherapy.
- Try sucking on ice chips; it may be soothing.

Some individuals find relief with a homemade gargle: Mix one-half teaspoon of salt and one teaspoon of baking soda in one quart of water, and gargle every four hours.

Hand-Foot Syndrome

Chemotherapy used for colorectal cancers may also cause a side effect called *hand-foot syndrome*. Symptoms typically show up in the hands and feet and include redness, swelling, blisters, and flaking skin. If symptoms become severe, they can impair walking and hand function. Your doctor will likely prescribe topical ointments for this condition. Here are other measures that may help:

- Limit use of hot water on hands and feet.
- Take cool baths.
- Pat skin dry after bathing; do not rub skin.
- Use ice packs for no more than fifteen minutes at a time. Never apply ice directly to skin—wrap the ice in a cloth.
- Apply skin-care creams as recommended by your doctor.
- Avoid exposure to direct sunlight.
- Moisturize a much as possible.

- Avoid activities, such as brisk exercise, that may cause clothing to rub against skin.

Although hand-foot syndrome typically affects hands and/or feet, it can also occur on the elbows and knees.

Rash

Another potential side effect of some chemotherapy is an acne-like rash, called *acneiform rash*. This rash may appear around the nose, or on the face, chest, or back. Interestingly, the rash is an indication that the chemotherapy is working. Your physician may prescribe antibiotics pills or topical gels to treat the rash. Over-the-counter medications to relieve itching may also be recommended.

Changes in Skin and Nails

Changes can occur in the skin and nails during chemotherapy. Skin reactions may include drying, cracking, or peeling. Also, skin may become *hyperpigmented,* meaning the skin may darken. This may happen all over the body or in spots, causing blotches and discoloration. When a change in skin color occurs, it usually appears about two to three weeks after chemotherapy treatment begins. When treatment ends, the discoloration usually goes away as new skin cells grow. Sometimes, however, the darkening is permanent. It's important to wear sunscreen when exposed to sunlight.

Nails may become discolored, and depressions may develop in both the fingernails and toenails. Once treatment is over and the nails resume normal growth, these depressions should disappear.

Allergic Reaction

An allergic reaction to a chemotherapy agent is not common, but it can occur. Symptoms of such a reaction include shortness of breath, wheezing, hoarseness, swelling, hives, and itching. These symptoms may occur within seconds of beginning a treatment, or they may occur a few hours or days later. More severe rare allergic reactions may lower blood pressure or cause heart attack, shock, or loss of consciousness. Medications can be given to counteract allergic reactions. If a reaction occurs outside your treatment center, you should contact your physician immediately.

Infertility

Colorectal cancer mostly affects men and women who are older and no longer in their childbearing years. However, when younger cancer patients undergo chemotherapy for colorectal cancer, their fertility can be affected. This side effect is rare, but it is possible for women to have damage to their ovaries, while men may suffer damage to the delicate lining of the testicles, where sperm is produced. Among those whose fertility is affected, some women and men are eventually able to conceive; others are not. You'll want to speak with your oncologist if infertility is an issue.

Damage to the Liver and Kidneys

Chemotherapy drugs may cause damage to the liver and kidneys. The liver's primary function is to filter toxic substances from the body. If the liver is damaged, these toxins can build up and cause more liver damage. However, after chemotherapy is stopped, other drugs can be given to lessen the effects of liver damage.

The kidneys filter waste from the blood. It's not common, but chemotherapy can damage the blood vessels in the kidneys, causing them to malfunction. This malfunction is called *acute renal failure*. Fortunately, kidney failure is usually reversible. When chemotherapy is stopped, other measures can be taken to clear toxins from the blood, allowing the kidneys time to recover.

Memory and Thinking Impairment

Some people have temporary changes in their memory or thinking process as side effects of chemotherapy. Sometimes referred to as "chemo brain" or "brain fog," these impairments are usually mild, but can be frustrating. You might feel confused, have problems concentrating, or have trouble finding the right word you want to use to express yourself. These side effects may linger for months or possibly years. The severity of such side effects depends on how much chemotherapy was given and the length of time it was given.

If you find yourself coping with this side effect, here are steps you can take:

- Keep a notepad handy to make notes to yourself.
- Keep a calendar nearby for scheduling events.
- Get plenty of rest.
- Ask for support from family members and friends.

Some patients use exercise, music therapy, art, and reading to help overcome the mental impairments; crossword puzzles and math games are also helpful in keeping your brain active.

Living with Chemotherapy Side Effects

As you read through the list of potential side effects, the idea of undergoing chemotherapy can be worrisome. However, most people tolerate chemotherapy with only mild to moderate side effects. Many colorectal cancer patients report that their chemotherapy was not as bad as they had thought it would be.

Targeted Therapy

Physicians and researchers have discovered that tumor types can differ in each person, depending on the cancer's genetic makeup and the molecules that are on a tumor's surface. *Targeted therapy* differs from chemotherapy because it mainly attacks cancer cells and does not affect normal cells as much. This generally means milder side effects compared to those resulting from chemotherapy. Targeted therapy may be given alone or along with chemotherapy.

How Targeted Therapy Works

Every single cell in our body constantly grows and changes. Our genes are in charge of ensuring that cells grow normally. Cancer cells grow in our bodies when genes change, or mutate, and make cells grow abnormally and out of control. Targeted therapies have been developed to pinpoint those changes and stop, or slow down, the cancerous growth. They attack the specific genes or proteins that create cancer cells.

The way cancer cells develop in one person may vary from the way it develops in another person. There is no one "switch" that controls all cancer cell growth. Accordingly, targeted therapies can work in a variety of ways. Some attack proteins or molecules inside cancer cells to stop the cells from reproducing. Some therapies stop the growth of cancer cells by targeting proteins on the surface of a cancer cell. Other targeted therapies affect how blood vessels grow so the tumors will have less blood and oxygen.

Many targetable mutations and proteins have been discovered for colorectal cancer. In some cases drugs have been developed to successfully attack those targets; in other cases a drug may not have been found to work. Research continues.

Are You a Candidate for Targeted Therapy?

In colorectal cancer, a patient's cancer tissue is tested to see if a targetable mutation or protein is present. A blood test, or a "liquid biopsy," may be used if a tissue sample isn't available. A liquid biopsy is a simple and noninvasive alternative to surgical biopsies that enables doctors to discover information about a tumor through a blood sample. Traces of a cancer's DNA in the blood can give clues about which treatments are most likely to work for a patient. The use of a targeted therapy is limited to those patients who have a mutation or specific protein.

A targeted treatment may be in a pill form which you can take at home, or given as an intravenous infusion in the cancer clinic. Targeted therapy can be given by itself, or with other chemotherapeutic agents.

Targeted Therapy Side Effects

Besides the possibility of a targeted therapy being more effective on one's cancer, the side effects tend to be milder than those of chemotherapy. Depending on the type of molecule your medicine is trying to target, general side effects can include upset stomach or diarrhea, skin rashes, liver function changes, fatigue, and headache. Rarer side effects include high blood pressure, bleeding (usually nosebleeds), clotting, or changes in sodium levels. It is important to note that many people on targeted therapy experience minimal side effects and tolerate the medications quite well. Your oncologist will let you know about any possible side effects of the drug you're taking.

Effectiveness of Targeted Therapy

Many patients with a diagnosis of colorectal cancer who receive targeted therapies will see a significant shrinkage of their tumor. The goals of treatment for these patients would be to control the disease for as long as possible. Studies have shown these drugs can prolong life by months to years. The reason a targeted therapy can stop working is similar to how chemotherapy may stop working—the cancer gets "smart." It can mutate or find a way to continue growing despite the medications. In these cases, the patient can be tested for new mutations or proteins. Based on the results a new drug, or a combination of drugs including chemotherapy, may be started.

Immunotherapy

Our immune system is our body's defense system against bacteria, viruses, and other foreign invaders. The immune response is a series of steps that stops substances from entering the body and causing sickness or disease. The immune system not only fights against infections, it also protects us from cancer cells. Immunotherapy uses our body's own immune system to fight cancer.

There are several types of immunotherapy, though all have the same goal: to use the immune system to fight diseases such as cancer. Some drugs stimulate our own immune system to work harder and attack cancer cells (these drugs are called *checkpoint inhibitors*).

Research shows that medicationscan be given to produce an immune response. Immunotherapy has been shown to work better for some cancer types than others, and it appears to be more effective if given with other types of treatment such chemotherapy or other immuno-therapies.

How Immunotherapy Works

Scientists have discovered one way a cancer cell escapes the body's immune response. The cancer develops a protein on its surface called *PD-L1 (programmed death-ligand 1)*. Quite simply, a cancer cell with PD-L1 on its surface can hide from the immune system and continue to grow.

Immunotherapy is designed to stop these PD-L1 proteins and stop cancer growth. When PD-L1 is blocked by the immunotherapy, the immune system is then able to fight the cancer cells. The PD-L1 protein can be blocked or overcome by the immune response in many different ways. Scientific research continues.

Are You a Candidate for Immunotherapy?

Most patients whose tumors have the PD-L1 proteins on the surface of the cancer cells are considered candidates for immunotherapy. In addition, immunotherapy has been approved for patients with metastatic colorectal cancer (cancer that has spread to other parts of the body) if the cancer has one of two specific genetic features and has progressed while on chemotherapy. The genetic features are *DNA-mismatch repair deficiency (MMR)* and *high microsatellite instability (MSI-H)*. If a person's colorectal cancer has these genetic changes, they are considered to be more responsive to immunotherapy.

Side Effects of Immunotherapy

Patients generally have fewer side effects from immunotherapy than from chemotherapy. Common side effects include fatigue, fever, chills, and weakness. However, immunotherapy, unlike chemotherapy, can also cause more-serious side effects at any point during the treatment. This is because it can cause inflammation of any organ in your body, the most common being the lungs, colon, and skin. Symptoms could include shortness of breath, cough, chest pain (if inflammation of the lungs), diarrhea (if inflammation of the colon), and rash (if inflammation of the skin). Side effects can affect the liver, pancreas, thyroid gland, and adrenal glands as well. Treatment of organ inflammation would generally be to hold the immunotherapy and start a short course of steroids. The decision to restart any immunotherapy would be a decision for your oncologist.

If you receive immunotherapy, it is important to know what to look for in terms of side effects, and call your physician at the first sign of any concerns. Research is being done to help identify who may respond to immunotherapy as well as who may experience side effects.

Effectiveness of Immunotherapy

Immunotherapy, like targeted therapy, is an evolving science. Scientists still need to learn why some patients respond to therapy as expected and some don't. At present, about 30 percent of patients with a

MSI-H genetic feature respond to immunotherapy. Some promising options are to combine immunotherapy and chemotherapy, combine immunotherapy and targeted therapy, or combine two different types of immunotherapy. As science progresses, oncologists will have a better understanding as to who will respond to immunotherapy and when to administer it.

6 RADIATION THERAPY

R adiation therapy is an important tool in treating many cancers, including colon and rectal cancers. Patients undergoing radiation therapy today benefit from far more-advanced medical technologies than were available a generation ago.

Sophisticated scanning devices produce multidimensional pictures that help doctors pinpoint the treatment area. State-of-the-art computers calculate and deliver radiation dosages so precisely that they destroy cancer cells but cause minimal damage to healthy tissues.

Radiation therapy is overseen by a *radiation oncologist,* a physician with specialty training in treating cancer with radiation. Other team members involved in treatment include: a *medical radiation physicist,* who ensures that radiation is properly tailored to each patient; a *medical dosimetrist,* who calculates the dosage; and a radiation therapist, who typically delivers the actual treatments.

How Radiation Therapy Works

Radiation kills cells that multiply rapidly. Because cancer cells multiply in a rapid, chaotic fashion, radiation treatments can stop them from reproducing. Healthy cells may also be affected by radiation, but they are not as vulnerable to it as are fast-growing cancer cells. The goal of radiation therapy is to eliminate cancer cells and spare the surrounding healthy cells; however, some damage to

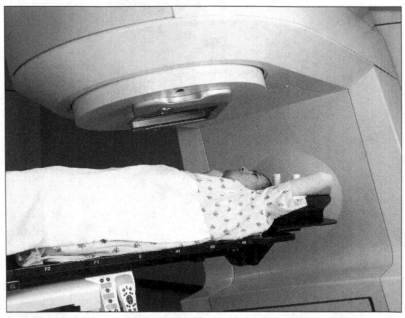

External beam radiation is delivered by a linear accelerator. Treatments are usually given five days a week over a period of five to eight weeks.

healthy tissues is often unavoidable. Fortunately, normal cells are able to repair themselves over time.

Radiation Therapy for Colon Cancer

Radiation therapy is occasionally used as a follow-up treatment after surgery for colon cancer, with the intention of killing any cancer cells that may remain after the removal of a primary tumor. Radiation therapy may also be recommended if the cancer has attached to a neighboring organ, such as the kidney, bladder, or spleen, or has infiltrated the lining of the abdomen. Postsurgical radiation therapy may also be combined with chemotherapy.

Radiation Therapy for Rectal Cancer

Radiation therapy plays a routine role in treating rectal cancer. Radiation is frequently used prior to surgery to shrink the tumor so it can be removed, and a colostomy can be avoided. (A colostomy is an external bag, worn to collect waste.) Shrinking the tumor first with radiation increases the chances of destroying the cancer completely. In fact, research shows that the risk of recurrence over the next ten years is cut by 50 percent when patients receive radiation therapy to the rectal area prior to surgery.

In addition, your doctor may recommend radiation therapy after surgery to kill any cancer cells that may remain.

Before Your First Treatment

Before your first radiation treatment, you will have a simulation appointment with your radiation therapy team. This is a planning session during which they will determine where the radiation beams will be directed and how your body will be positioned for each treatment.

During the simulation, you'll be asked to lie on a treatment table, either on your stomach or on your back. You'll be fitted with an immobilization device; it is a comfortable, yet rigid, cradle that holds your body in place during each treatment session. The immobilization device is created by pouring resin or polystyrene beads into a bag made of urethane, nylon, or another sturdy material. The bag is then molded to the specific contours of your body.

You will be given a contrast fluid—you will either be given an injection or will be asked to drink a solution with the contrast. This contrast will show up in tissues when you undergo a body scan. This scan, which gives your doctor a detailed view of the tumor and the surrounding healthy tissues, pinpoints the part of the body to be treated.

After the treatment area is defined and filmed, a technologist will mark your skin with tiny, permanent tattoos. These tiny marks serve as a "map" that tells the radiation therapist where to direct the radiation beam during treatments. (The tattoos appear as tiny freckles and most patients do not find them bothersome.)

Receiving a Radiation Treatment

During a treatment, you lie on a treatment table while the arm of the linear accelerator circles your body, sending calculated radiation doses to the tumor.

External beam radiation therapy is typically administered five days a week over five to eight weeks. Each treatment lasts a few minutes, but the preparation takes longer. The treatments are spread over time because the total dosage necessary to kill a tumor would cause too much damage to normal tissues if given at once. You need time for your healthy cells to repair themselves.

Types of Radiation Therapy

There are several types of radiation that may be used to treat colon and rectal cancer. These range from external beams of radiation that are aimed at your tumor, to internal treatments, in which the radiation is aimed at internal cancerous tissues. Your radiation oncologist will discuss with you the best type of radiation for you.

The most common radiation treatment option for colon and rectal cancer is *external beam radiation therapy,* or *EBRT.* This type of treatment sends radiation rays into a tumor from outside the body. A high-energy X-ray unit called a *linear accelerator (LINAC),* generates the beams, which target the tumor while sparing internal tissues and skin.

Three-Dimensional Conformal Radiation Therapy

A type of external beam radiation therapy, *three-dimensional conformal radiation therapy (3D-CRT)* is an advanced technology used in many medical facilities to treat colon and rectal cancers. It involves the use of special CT scanners and computers to map the tumor in three-dimensional form and then match, or conform, beams to the cancer's unique shape. Once the outline is calculated, the radiation is aimed at the tumor from multiple angles.

A specialized form of conformal radiation therapy, known as *intensity modulated radiation therapy (IMRT)*, may be used. In addition to conforming radiation beams to an individual mass, IMRT allows radiation oncologists to break up each beam into smaller "beamlets" and adjust them in intensity, or strength. With such capability, doctors can deliver an even higher dose of radiation to the tumor while minimizing damage to nearby healthy tissues. Although IMRT is offered at many medical centers, some insurers won't cover the cost.

Image-Guided Radiation Therapy

Another form of radiation treatment, *image-guided radiation therapy (IGRT)*, uses images, such as X-rays or CT scans, to help radiation oncologists deliver the radiation beam more precisely. Because tumors and healthy tissues can shift between treatments, viewing these areas allows physicians to make corrections and tailor the beam's focus. During IGRT, the doctor "fuses" the images during your simulation session with new images taken that day, to see if adjustments must be made. Available at many medical centers, IGRT is used to treat both colon and rectal cancers.

Intraoperative Radiation Therapy

During surgery, another form of radiation treatment, *intraoperative radiation therapy (IORT)*, is used to deliver a dose of intense radiation to a tumor or to an area at risk of tumor recurrence. After the surgeon removes as much of the mass as possible, a linear accelerator delivers a concentrated, high-dose beam directly to the remaining part of the tumor or the area from which the tumor has been removed. Although IORT shows promise for colon and anal cancers, the technology is not commonly used.

It's currently available at only a few medical centers. In these locations, it's used to treat malignancies that either are attached to vital tissues or can't be removed entirely. The treatment is also effective for tumors that can't be cured with surgery alone or that will likely regrow in the same area.

Internal Radiation Therapy

Internal radiation therapy, also called *brachythera-py,* involves the use of radioactive pellets that are inserted next to or directly into a tumor. Although brachytherapy has a limited role in treating colon cancer, it's used somewhat routinely in treating rectal cancer.

Endocavitary radiation therapy, a specialized form of brachytherapy, is effective in the treatment of small, early-stage rectal cancers. In this procedure, a high dose of radiation is administered through the rectum with a device that is inserted into the rectum for each treatment; it is removed after the treatment. The advantage of this endocavitary approach is that the radiation reaches the rectum without passing through the skin or tissues of the abdomen.

The patient is usually awake during these radiation treatments, which take about twenty minutes each. The treatment is repeated several times over several weeks. The procedure is usually performed at larger hospitals but may also be offered at some community hospitals.

Side Effects of Radiation Therapy

Radiation treatments are not painful—most patients don't feel anything during a radiation treatment. Yet the beams can affect any skin, muscle, and abdominal organs in its path. This can produce symptoms ranging from skin irritation to the irradiated area to changes in bowel movements. Although side effects can be distressing, most symptoms are treatable. They usually disappear after therapy, although some symptoms may be permanent.

Also, keep in mind that not everyone experiences every side effect.

Skin Irritation

Skin irritation is the most common side effect of radiation therapy. As treatment progresses, any skin in the beam's path may become dry, irritated, and peel like a sunburn. The changes may leave the skin rough and darkened. You can minimize any irritation during treatment, however, by taking these measures:

- Wear loose, soft clothing over the treated area.
- Avoid any lotion, soap, or powder on the area within four hours just before treatment.
- Ask your doctor or nurse about lotions or creams that may help after treatment.
- Avoid rubbing, scratching, or scrubbing the treated skin.
- Bathe in lukewarm water.

Loss of Appetite

Because the beams can be hard on the lining of your gastrointestinal tract, radiation can affect your appetite, particularly if you're being treated for colon cancer. Rectal cancer patients usually don't experience a loss of appetite. In either case, however, it's important to maintain a nutritious diet so your body will stay energized. If you lose your appetite, here are some suggestions to follow:

- Eat smaller, more-frequent meals, including healthful snacks.
- Avoid fatty foods.
- Work with a dietitian to develop a plan that helps you maintain or gain weight.

Diarrhea and Nausea

Diarrhea is a common side effect of radiation therapy for both colon and rectal cancer. Because the bowel and stomach are sensitive to radiation, they may become inflamed, triggering abdominal symptoms. You may experience bloating, cramps, and chronic diarrhea, or frequent bowel movements. If you're undergoing treatment for colon cancer, you may also have bouts of nausea. Fortunately, by being proactive, you can alleviate such symptoms. In the case of diarrhea, follow these measures:

- Increase your intake of fluids, such as broth. Drink at least six eight-ounce glasses of fluids daily; persistent diarrhea can cause your body to lose water and nutrients.

- Avoid caffeine (such as coffee and tea) and alcohol-containing drinks, because they lead to fluid loss.

- Avoid foods that intensify diarrhea: milk products, nuts, seeds, raw high-fiber vegetables (such as corn, cauliflower, and broccoli), and fruits with skins.

- Choose foods low in fiber, such as bananas, applesauce, rice, and toast.

- Try drinking ginger tea or eating ginger candy.

- Tell your doctor if you have watery, loose stools more than two or three times a day or notice mucus or blood in the stool.

- If you have diarrhea, your doctor may prescribe an antidiarrheal medication. Don't take over-the-counter medications without consulting your physician.

You can minimize nausea by avoiding sweet, fried, spicy, or fatty foods and substituting bland items, such as dry crackers and flat ginger ale. It helps to eat smaller, more frequent meals. Also, eat foods at room temperature if the odor of hot foods upsets your stomach. Other tips include:

- Breathe deeply and slowly when you feel nauseous.
- Learn relaxation exercises to help you feel less anxious and more in control.
- Ask your doctor about medications or other devices, such as wrist acupressure bands, that may decrease the problem.

Bowel function usually returns to normal after treatment is completed. However, some people notice more frequent bowel movements and/or loose stools after radiation treatment; these changes can last indefinitely.

Bladder Irritation

Because the bladder is close to the rectum, radiation therapy may affect this organ, potentially causing infection, burning when urinating, or even blood in the urine. You may feel like you have to urinate when you really don't need to. Bladder irritation is rarely a permanent side effect.

Rectal Irritation

When radiation is directed at a rectal tumor, inflammation is a common side effect. You may experience itching or burning pain during bowel movements. Your rectum also may be sore if your bowels are moving frequently. In either case, there are steps you can take to relieve the discomfort:

- Take sitz baths—sit in a few inches of warm water.
- Pat your rectal area dry with a soft cloth after cleansing.
- Ask your doctor about safe and effective creams and suppositories.

The affected area should heal after treatment has ended. Permanent rectal discomfort can occur, but it's infrequent.

Fatigue

Many patients report being tired during radiation therapy, particularly as the treatments progress. Treatment takes time, during which your energy levels may be lower than normal. Such fatigue is more common when you receive chemotherapy along with radiation. However, the fatigue should diminish within weeks of finishing treatment. Until then, you can counter your low energy by following these suggestions:

- Take short rests when you feel tired. Avoid long naps so you sleep well at night, and move slowly when you lie down or sit up to avoid dizziness.

- Do mild exercise; add a brisk twenty-minute walk to your daily routine.

- Take in sufficient calories; poor eating habits can add to fatigue, but a healthful diet can help immeasurably.

- Drink plenty of liquids; drinking six to eight glasses of water daily helps you stay hydrated and energized as well.

During treatment, it's also a good idea to focus on important tasks. If your fatigue is severe or chronic, ask for help with routine daily chores or prioritize what needs to be done.

Infections

Radiation can cause a reduction in your white blood cell count. (White blood cells fight infection.) This effect is much more likely, however, when radiation and chemotherapy are delivered at the same time. Without sufficient white blood cells, your body can't fight infections adequately. Because it's important to stay healthy during your therapy, be sure to take these measures:

- Wash your hands often to kill germs.
- Avoid people with colds, and avoid crowds. Also avoid children who've been recently vaccinated with live viruses.
- Protect yourself against cuts and open sores that could become infected.
- Call your doctor immediately if you develop any signs of an infection: severe chills, a cough, a temperature of 100.5°F or higher, or pain during urination.

Whatever your side effects might be from radiation therapy, it's important to remember that they can be managed, if not eliminated completely. With guidance from your medical team, you can address most of the problems successfully.

Living with Radiation Therapy Side Effects

Side effects of radiation therapy for colon and rectal cancers can be managed. Still, it is important to be aware of the side effects that you may experience so you can report them to your oncologist. The sooner your physician knows about side effects, the sooner he or she can take steps to alleviate them.

7 FOLLOW-UP CARE

After you've been treated for colorectal cancer, your physician will monitor you closely for any signs of cancer recurrence. You will be scheduled for periodic examinations for the next few years.

Follow-up treatment typically involves examinations every three to six months for the first two to three years, and then every six months for the next two years. If you have been treated for an early-stage cancer, you may not require monitoring as frequently. Follow-up examinations will include several diagnostic tests.

Diagnostic Tests

The tests you'll undergo as part of your follow-up care are the same types of diagnostic tests you had prior to your treatment. They involve blood tests, X-rays, scans, and colonoscopies.

Blood Tests

Routine blood tests may also measure your levels of a protein called *carcinoembryonic antigen (CEA)*—often referred to as a *tumor marker*. These markers are chemicals made by tumor cells and can be detected in your blood. Doctors test the levels of these markers prior to treatment and usually find that elevated levels go down after treatment. However, if levels go back up, it may be a sign that the cancer has recurred. If your doctor finds high levels of CEA, he or she will perform other tests to inves-

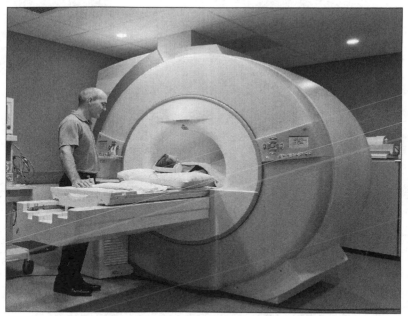

As part of follow-up care, your physician may schedule CT scans annually for the first three years after your treatment.

tigate further, probably with routine blood tests, every three months for the first three years after your treatment.

Note that elevated levels of these tumor markers in the blood does *not* always mean cancer has recurred. Increased levels may also be symptoms of noncancerous conditions, such as gallstones, rectal polyps, inflammation, cirrhosis, peptic ulcers, pancreatitis, ulcerative colitis, emphysema, or benign breast disease.

Imaging Tests

Imaging tests allow your physician to view your internal organs. Such tests may include CT scans, PET scans, MRI scans, bone scans, or ultrasound scans. If your doctor determines that you have a higher risk for colon cancer recurrence, he or she may schedule routine scans of your chest and abdomen. If there is a risk for recurrence of rectal cancer, your physician will likely schedule scans of your pelvis. These tests are typically recommended once a year for the first three years.

Colonoscopy

Your physician will want you to have regular colonoscopies that will check for polyps or any new tumors. A colonoscopy is usually recommended in the first year after surgery, then once every three years. If these tests show no signs of cancer, the next colonoscopy is usually recommended at five years. The frequency of the colonoscopies is related to the nature of your risk for recurrence.

Cancer Recurrence

What if the cancer recurs? This is the question that lingers in the minds of most cancer patients and their families. Your risk of recurrence is directly related to the stage of your cancer at the time of the initial diagnosis. A cancer caught early and confined to the colorectal wall is less likely to recur than a cancer that has spread to surrounding tissue or lymph nodes at the time of initial diagnosis.

If colorectal cancer recurs, it usually does so within the first five years after diagnosis and treatment. Recurrent cancer is divided into three categories. When cancer recurs very near the same site as the original cancer, it is called a *local recurrence*. It is a *regional recurrence* if the cancer is found in lymph nodes and tissues near the original site. If the cancer recurs in other parts of the body, it is considered a *distant recurrence*. The liver is the most common organ in which colorectal cancer recurs.

Once you've finished your initial treatments and it's time to see your physician for a follow-up examination, you may be anxious, especially in the beginning; however, most people report that they become less anxious as time goes on.

Symptoms of Cancer Recurrence

It is important to stay alert for any symptoms of cancer recurrence so that it can be diagnosed and treated early. The symptoms of a recurring colorectal cancer are similar to the symptoms of an initial colorectal cancer.

- *Change in bowel habits:* Prolonged constipation not responsive to laxatives, abdominal pain, persistent diarrhea, or a change in stool characteristics.

- *Rectal bleeding:* Passing dark or bright red blood with bowel movements, or a change in stool color.

- *Persistent urge to have a bowel movement:* Urge to have a bowel movement despite just having had a bowel movement.

- *Excess mucus secretion:* With bowel movements.

- *Chronic abdominal pain, bloating, and fullness:* Persistent discomfort that does not go away with medications.

- *Decreased appetite, weight loss, and fatigue:* Possible signs of a recurrence in the liver or other organs.

- *Jaundice:* A yellowing of the eyes or skin, which may indicate a recurrence in the liver.

- *New joint or bone pain:* Onset of acute back or rib pain may be a symptom of a recurrence in the spine.

Treatment for Recurring Cancer

Options for treating colorectal cancer that returns include: surgery, chemotherapy, radiation therapy, or a combination of these treatments. Other potential treatments include various liver-directed therapies to any cancer that has spread to the liver. These can include chemotherapy infusions directly into the blood supplying the liver as well as cryoablations and radiofrequency ablations. Treatment with cryoablation involves freezing cancerous tissue with liquid nitrogen. Radiofrequency ablation involves applying intense heat to cancerous cells.

Clinical Trials

Your oncologist may recommend participation in a clinical trial. These trials may be part of a person's initial treatment. Or, they may be recommended after standard treatments have failed. A clinical trial is a research study, conducted with patients, that applies new treatments or new combinations of treatments to those chosen to participate. Many of today's best standard treatments were first available to patients in clinical trials.

It is important to remember that participants in clinical trials do *not* receive untested treatments. Participants are not treated as "human guinea pigs." New treatments are offered to patients in clinical trials only after extensive laboratory research has demonstrated that these treatments are at least as good as, and potentially much better than, standard therapies.

Participating in a Clinical Trial

Participation in a clinical trial is strictly voluntary. You may stop participating in a clinical trial at any time before, during, or after you have received the new treatment. Upon leaving the trial, if any medical problems result from the trial treatment, you will continue to receive appropriate medical care.

How do you enroll in a trial? Researchers set guidelines for who is eligible to participate in a clinical trial. These guidelines include factors such as age, sex, type and stage of disease, previous treatment history, and other medical conditions. Ask your doctor or oncologist to help you find a trial that is suitable. He or she will ask you to sign a consent form after reviewing all the details of the clinical trial with you, including the potential benefits and risks.

98

Benefits and Risks of Clinical Trials

There are potential benefits and risks to participating in a clinical trial. The National Cancer Institute lists the benefits and risks as follows:

Potential Benefits

- Health care is provided by leading physicians in the field of cancer research.

- You receive access to new drugs and interventions before they are widely available.

- Your health is closely monitored.

- You have a more active role in your own health care.

- If the approach being studied is found to be helpful, you may be among the first to benefit.

- The trial is an opportunity to make a valuable contribution to cancer research.

Potential Risks

- Despite research on new drugs and procedures, it's possible that the treatments may have side effects or risks unknown to the doctors.

- New drugs and procedures may be ineffective or may be less effective than current approaches.

- Even if a new approach has benefits, it may not work for you.

Where to Find Clinical Trials

Clinical trials are offered in hospitals, cancer centers, doctors' offices, and clinics throughout the United States and internationally. However, some trials are available only at certain locations. Clinical trials are sponsored by a number of organizations, both public and private. The National Cancer Institute sponsors many clinical trials and works with other organizations that sponsor clinical trials. You'll find website information about the National Cancer Institute in the Resources section at the back of this book.

8 PREVENTION AND EARLY DETECTION

Studies have repeatedly shown that annual screening for colorectal cancer prolongs survival and saves lives. In fact, annual screening actually reduces your risk of getting colorectal cancer by up to 20 percent—when precancerous polyps are found, they can be removed before they become cancerous. Unfortunately, today only about 40 percent of Americans undergo any type of routine screening. As a result, colorectal cancer remains the third leading cause of cancer death in the United States.

Screening According to Risk Factors

How often should you be screened for colorectal cancer? The frequency of screening depends on whether you have an average, increased, or high risk for developing the disease. Those in the average risk category are those with no known risk factors; this includes nearly 75 percent of Americans.

Average Risk

If you are at average risk, you should start undergoing routine screening once you reach the age of forty-five. The following screening tests are recommended:

- A fecal occult blood test every year. This test checks for hidden blood in stool samples.

- A flexible sigmoidoscopy every five years. This test examines the interior walls of the rectum and the lower third of the colon. The majority of cancers start in this area.
- A colonoscopy every ten years. This test examines the entire length of the colon.

Increased Risk

Individuals are considered at increased risk if they have a history of polyps that can become cancerous; have had colon or rectal cancer; have a first-degree relative (parent, brother, sister, or child) who has had colorectal cancer or polyps; or have two or more second-degree relatives (aunt, uncle, grandparent) who have had colorectal cancer. These are the recommendations for screening:

- Colonoscopy is the only screening test that should be recommended.
- In the case of a family history of cancer or polyps in a first-degree relative, your first colonoscopy should be done at age forty or ten years earlier than the age of the youngest relative when he or she was diagnosed with colorectal cancer. For example, if your father was diagnosed with colorectal cancer at age forty-five, you should begin having routine colonoscopies at age thirty-five.

Colonoscopy recommendations for individuals at increased risk of colorectal cancer vary based on factors such as how many polyps they have and the size of the polyps. If you're in this group, talk with your doctor about when to begin colonoscopy screening and how often it should be repeated.

High Risk

You are considered at high risk for colorectal cancer if you have a personal history of inflammatory bowel disease, including Crohn's disease and ulcerative colitis, of sufficient duration—at least eight years. You are also at high risk if you have a family history of hereditary colorectal cancer. The two types of this cancer are familial adenomatous polyposis (FAP) and hereditary nonpolyposis colorectal cancer (HNPCC), discussed in chapter 1.

If you are at high risk, talk to your doctor about how often you should be screened. The frequency of screening depends on the type of risk factor you have. Here are the guidelines:

- If you have inflammatory bowel disease, Crohn's disease, or ulcerative colitis, routine colonoscopies are recommended every one to two years. Talk with your doctor about how soon after the onset of the disease you should start the colonoscopies. Also ask about undergoing a tissue biopsy to check for any abnormal cells in the lining of the colon.

- If you have familial adenomatous polypsis, get a flexible sigmoidoscopy or colonoscopy every six to twelve months once you reach puberty.

- If you have hereditary nonpolyposis colon cancer syndrome, experts recommend a colonoscopy every two years starting at age twenty-five. This should continue until you reach age forty. Thereafter, schedule a colonoscopy every year.

Genetic Testing

An estimated 5 to 10 percent of all colorectal cancers involve inherited genes. If you have a strong family history of colorectal cancer, such as several members diagnosed before age sixty, genetic tests are now available that can predict your risk of developing the disease later in life.

These genetic tests involve sampling your blood to test for gene mutations, which are abnormal genes. If you test positive for these genetic mutations, you have an 80 percent higher risk than the average person of developing colorectal cancer as you get older. If you have familial adenomatous polyposis or hereditary nonpolyposis colorectal cancer, you have a 50 percent chance of passing the abnormal gene on to each of your children.

By knowing your risk, you and your doctor can develop an aggressive screening program that can detect cancer early or prevent it altogether.

Lifestyle Factors and Colorectal Cancer

Several lifestyle factors can influence the development of colorectal cancer. These factors include diet, body weight, exercise, smoking, and the use of supplements and medications.

Proper Nutrition

Diet plays a major role in our health. Some studies show that diet is a factor in the development of colorectal cancer. It is well known that colorectal cancer is primarily a disease of Western industrialized countries such as the United States and Canada. The lifetime risk of getting the disease in Western countries is 6 percent, but the incidence is much lower in countries such as Japan, where much less red meat and fat are consumed. According to some studies, by adhering to a healthful diet, you can reduce your risk of colorectal cancer by up to 50 percent.

Reducing your intake of processed and red meat, cholesterol, and saturated fatty acids can help prevent precancerous polyps and colorectal cancer. A diet high in fruits and vegetables may also help prevent the formation of polyps and cancer. Fruits and green, leafy vegetables contain antioxidants that protect cells against cancer-causing agents in our diet and in the environment. Antioxidants include vitamins A, C, and E. Carotenoids, lycopene, and lutein are other antioxidants commonly found in fruits and vegetables.

It's also believed that fiber helps prevent colorectal cancer. Fiber promotes good bowel function, dilutes carcinogens in our diet that ultimately make their way to the colon, and decreases the time the inner lining of the colon is exposed to carcinogens.

Some studies have suggested that a diet deficient in calcium increases your risk of developing polyps and colorectal cancer. One study showed a 20 percent reduction in the incidence of colorectal cancer in patients taking calcium supplements. Calcium appears to block the effects of some carcinogens found in the colon and helps prevent polyp and cancer formation. Vitamin D may also help guard against colorectal cancer since it helps the body absorb calcium.

Alcohol consumption may also be a factor in the development of colorectal cancer. It's believed that consuming more than three alcoholic drinks a day increases the risk of forming large polyps.

Body Weight and Exercise

Obesity is linked to colorectal cancer in both men and women, but the link seems to be stronger in men. Some studies show that carrying extra fat around the waist increases the risk of colorectal cancer.

Studies also confirm the benefits of daily vigorous exercise in preventing colorectal cancer. Daily exercise is helpful in preventing many other diseases as well, such as heart and lung disease. Try to get at least thirty minutes of exercise, such as brisk walking, every day.

Smoking

It's a fact that smoking causes lung cancer, and it may also contribute to other cancers, including colorectal cancer. As technology to analyze the DNA in genes becomes more advanced, the link between smoking and colorectal cancer becomes stronger. Medical data suggests that smoking can have a damaging effect on the DNA of colon cells, predisposing them to becoming cancerous. By smoking, you increase your risk for a number of noncancerous diseases as well. If you smoke, talk with your doctor about strategies to quit, including the use of prescription drugs and nicotine patches.

Hormone Therapy

There is emerging evidence that postmenopausal women who take the hormone supplements estrogen and progesterone have a reduced risk of getting colon cancer; however, estrogen alone does not appear to reduce the risk. This evidence comes mainly from the millions of postmenopausal women who take hormone supplements to reduce the risk of osteoporosis—weakening of the bones. However, research also links hormone therapy to heart disease, blood clots, and breast, lung, and uterine cancers.

The hormones estrogen and progesterone do not appear to lower the risk for rectal cancer.

Aspirin and Other Medications

Aspirin and similar medications can prevent the formation of polyps and colorectal cancer. Over the last three decades, several large studies have focused on people taking an aspirin a day to reduce the risk of heart disease. Surprisingly, these studies show that individuals who have taken aspirin daily for at least five years also have a 40 to 50 percent reduction in the risk of polyps and colorectal cancer. Researchers believe that aspirin somehow reverses the precancerous changes in growing precancerous polyps.

Other aspirin-like medications, including ibuprofen, have the same effect. Ibuprofen is a nonsteroidal anti-inflammatory drug (NSAID) and is primarily used to treat pain and inflammation. However, these medications also carry side effects such as possible bleeding. Ask your doctor whether you should be taking any of them.

Importance of Early Detection

As mentioned earlier, the key to prevention and early detection of colorectal cancer is routine screening. The earlier colorectal cancer is diagnosed, the better the chance for a cure. Symptoms of an early colorectal cancer may be subtle or not noticeable at all. However, in cases that are diagnosed early, the cure rate is approximately 90 percent. Talk to your doctor about routine screenings.

Appendix

Simplified Summary of TNM Staging System for Colon and Rectal Cancer

The TNM staging system below is used by physicians to describe how far a cancer has spread. In the initials, TNM, the **T** stands for tumor—its size and the extent of any spreading. The **N** is for lymph nodes and refers to any spread of the cancer to lymph nodes. The **M** is for metastasis or spread to other organs The system will appear complex; you may wish to ask your doctor to help you understand it.

Tumor (T)	
Tx	Primary tumor cannot be assessed
T0	No evidence of primary tumor
Tis	Carcinoma *in situ:* Intraepithelial or invasion of lamina propria
T1	Tumor invades submucosa
T2	Tumor invades muscularis propria
T3	Tumor invades through the muscularis propria into pericolorectal tissues
T4a	Tumor penetrates to the surface of the visceral peritoneum
T4b	Tumor directly invades or is adherent to other organs and structures

Nodes (N)	
NX	Regional lymph nodes cannot be assessed
N0	No regional lymph node metastasis
N1	Metastasis in one to three regional lymph nodes
N1a	Metastasis in one regional lymph node
N1b	Metastasis in two to three regional lymph nodes
N1c	Tumor deposit(s) in the subserosa, mesentery, or nonperitonealized pericolic or perirectal tissues without regional nodal metastasis
N2	Metastasis in four or more regional lymph nodes
N2a	Metastasis in four to six regional lymph nodes
N2b	Metastasis in seven or more regional lymph nodes
Metastasis	
M0	No distant metastasis
M1	Distant metastasis
M1a	Metastasis confined to one organ or site (for example, liver, lung, ovary, nonregional node)
M1b	Metastasis in more than one organ/site or the peritoneum

Cancer Stages with TNM Classifications

Stage	T	N	M
0	Tis	N0	M0
I	T1	N0	M0
	T2	N0	M0
IIA	T3	N0	M0
IIB	T4a	N0	M0
IIC	T4b	N0	M0
IIIA	T1-2	N1/N1c	M0
	T1	N2a	M0
IIIB	T3-T4a	N1/N1c	M0
	T2-T3	N2a	M0
	T1-T2	N2b	M0
IIIC	T4a	N2a	M0
	T3-T4a	N2b	M0
	T4b	N1-N2	M0
IVA	Any T	Any N	M1a
IVB	Any T	Any N	M2b

Resources

American Cancer Society
15999 Clifton Road NE
Atlanta, GA 30329-4251
Phone: (800) 227-2345
www.cancer.org

American College of Gastroenterology
6400 Goldsboro Road, Suite 200
Bethesda, MD 20817
Phone: (301) 263-9000
www.gi.org

American College of Surgeons
633 North Saint Clair Street
Chicago, IL 60611
Phone: (312) 202-5000
www.facs.org

American Gastroenterological Association
4930 Del Ray Avenue
Bethesda, MD 20814
Phone: (301) 654-2055
www.gastro.org

American Society of Colon & Rectal Surgeons
85 West Algonquin Road, Suite 550
Arlington Heights, IL 60005
Phone: (847) 290-9184
www.fascrs.org

Cancer Care
275 7th Avenue
New York, NY 10001
Phone: (800) 813-HOPE (4673)
www.cancercare.org

Colon Cancer Challenge Foundation
10 New King Street, Suite 202
White Plains, NY 10604
Phone: (914) 305-6674
www.coloncancerchallenge.org

Colorectal Cancer Alliance
1025 Vermont Avenue NW, Suite 1066
Washington, DC 20005
Phone: (877) 442-2030
www.ccalliance.org

National Cancer Institute
9609 Medical Center Drive
Bethesda, MD 20892
Phone: (800) 422-6237 (4-CANCER)
www.cancer.gov

National Coalition for Cancer Survivorship
8455 Colesville Road, Suite 930
Silver Spring, MD 20910
Phone: (877) 622-7937
www.canceradvocacy.org

National Comprehensive Cancer Network
275 Commerce Drive, Suite 300
Fort Washington, PA 19034
Phone: (215) 690-0300
www.nccn.org

United Ostomy Associations of America, Inc.
P.O. Box 525
Kennebank, ME 04043
Phone: (800) 826-0826
www.ostemy.org

Wound Ostomy and Continence Nurses Society (WOCN)
1120 Route 73, Suite 200
Mount Laurel, NJ 08054
Phone: (888) 224-9626
www.wocn.org

GLOSSARY

A

acneiform rash: An acne-like reaction to some chemotherapy agents. Unlike true acne, the breakouts are sterile and contain no bacteria.

adenocarcinoma: The most common type of colorectal cancer.

adenoma: A benign glandular tumor which over time may become malignant.

adjuvant therapy: Additional therapy given to supplement an initial therapy.

ambulatory infusion pump: A small, wearable pump that delivers measured amounts of a drugs over time.

anemia: A medical term given to the condition of a low red blood cell count.

anesthesiologist: A doctor trained in administering anesthesia during surgery.

anterior-posterior (AP) resection: The major curative operation for cancers of the distal rectum.

anus: The opening at the end of the rectum where stool exits the body.

ascending colon: The first part of the colon on the right side of the abdominal cavity.

B

bacteremia: An infection of the blood stream caused by bacteria.

barium enema: An X-ray test that outlines the colon wall and is used to identify polyps.

benign: Noncancerous.

bilirubin: A compound made by the liver and involved in digestion of food.

biopsy: A procedure to surgically remove a piece of tissue for analysis.

bladder: The organ, located behind the pubic bone, that collects urine.

bone scan: A specialized X-ray test used to evaluate the skeleton for the spread of cancer.

brachytherapy: A form of radiation therapy used to treat cancer.

C

carcinoembryonic antigen (CEA): A protein in the blood specifically produced by cancer cells in the colon, rectum, pancreas, and breast.

carcinoma *in situ:* Cells that show the earliest signs of cancerous changes.

cecum: The beginning part of the right or ascending colon.

chemotherapy: Therapy that uses chemical agents to treat cancer.

colectomy: Surgery to remove all or some portion of the colon.

colon: The organ in the body responsible for the excretion of waste.

colonoscope: A fiber-optic, flexible scope used to perform a colonoscopy.

colonoscopy: The procedure doctors perform to examine the inside of the colon.

colorectal surgeon: A surgeon specifically trained to treat diseases of the colon and rectum.

colostomy: The sewing of an open end of colon to the skin on the abdomen so stool can flow into an attached, plastic pouch.

colostomy takedown: The reversal of colostomy, in which the large intestine is reconnected with the rectum to restore normal movement of stool.

complete blood count (CBC): A blood test used to measure the red and white blood cells in the body.

computerized axial tomography (CAT or CT) scan: A specialized X-ray used to examine the internal organs.

contrast: A liquid taken by mouth or injected into a vein to enhance the quality of X-ray pictures.

Cowden disease: An inherited disease resulting in the formation of colorectal polyps.

Crohn's disease: An inflammatory disease of the colon wall resulting in diarrhea and pain.

cryoablation: A process that uses extreme cold to remove tissue.

CT colonography: Often referred to as a virtual colonoscopy, a CT scan designed to simulate a colonoscopy to look for polyps and cancers.

cystogram: An X-ray test used to evaluate the inside lining of the bladder.

D

descending colon: The part of the colon located on the left side of the abdominal cavity and connecting to the sigmoid colon.

diarrhea: The passing of liquid stool.

diverticulosis: A disease of the colon characterized by the formation of small, weak pouches in the wall and resulting in constipation and pain.

duodenum: The name given to the first part of the small intestine leading from the stomach.

dysplastic: Precancerous changes seen in colorectal polyps.

E

electrolytes: Blood components of sodium, potassium, chloride, and carbon dioxide.

endocavitary radiation: A type of radiation treatment used to treat cancer.

enterostomal nurse: A nurse specializing in the education about and care of a colostomy.

epidural catheter: A small tube inserted at the base of the back for pain control after an operation.

esophagus: A tubelike organ that carries food from the mouth to the stomach.

external beam: A type of radiation treatment used to treat cancer.

extramural: Referring to outside the wall of an organ.

117

F

familial adenomatous polyposis (FAP): An inherited disease resulting in the formation of hundreds or thousands of precancerous polyps at an early age.

fatigue: Tiredness.

fecal occult blood test (FOBT): Checks for hidden blood in the stool.

fistula: An abnormal connection between two or more hollow organs.

forceps: A surgical instrument used to grab objects.

G

Gardner's syndrome: An inherited disease resulting in the formation of precancerous colorectal polyps.

gastroenterologist: A doctor specializing in treating diseases of the esophagus, stomach, intestine, colon, rectum, and anus.

gastrointestinal tract: An all-encompassing term given to the organs involved in eating, digestion, absorption, and waste excretion.

general anesthesia: Anesthesia given with the purpose of putting patients to sleep during surgery.

general surgeon: A surgeon qualified to operate on a variety of diseases, including colorectal cancer.

H

hamartoma polyp: A benign tumor that grows at the same rate as the surrounding tissue, but grows in a disorganized mass.

hand-foot syndrome: Side effect caused be chemotherapy agents leaking through veins and injuring tissues, often in the hands and feet.

hematocrit: Red blood cell count given as a percentage.

hemoglobin: The level of iron present as it relates to red blood cell count.

hemorrhoids: Abnormal veins located around the anus, causing bleeding and pain.

hepatic artery infusion: Delivers chemotherapeutic agents directly to the liver through a catheter placed in the hepatic artery.

hereditary nonpolyposis colorectal cancer (HNPCC): A hereditary disease resulting in the formation of one to five precancerous polyps at an early age.

hyperplastic polyp: A noncancerous polyp.

I

image-guided radiation therapy (IGRT): The use of frequent imaging during a course of radiation therapy to improve the precision and accuracy of the delivery of treatment.

immunotherapy: Uses the body's own immune system to fight cancer

incentive spirometer: A plastic device that patients blow into after surgery to keep their lungs expanded and prevent pneumonia.

incision: The surgical site where the actual cutting was performed during surgery.

inflammatory bowel disease (IBD): A disease characterized by inflammation of the lining or the entire wall of the colon.

inflammatory polyp: Growths which occur with acute or chronic inflammation.

intensity modulated radiation therapy (IMRT): A mode of high-precision radiotherapy that uses computer-controlled linear accelerators to deliver precise radiation doses to a tumor or specific areas within the tumor.

internal radiation therapy: A form a treatment in which a source of radiation is placed inside the body.

intraoperative radiation therapy (IORT): An intensive radiation treatment that delivers a concentrated beam of radiation to tumors as they are located during surgery.

intravenous: Refers to inside the vein. Many medications are given this way.

J

jaundice: A yellowing color of the skin or eyes as a result of a rise in the bilirubin level.

K

KRAS: A protein involved in cell division. The official name is v-Ki-ras2 Kirsten rat sarcoma viral oncogene homolog.

L

laparoscopic surgery: Surgery performed using small incisions and small instruments.

linear accelerator (LINAC): A device that creates the X-ray beams used during radiation therapy.

liver: The largest organ in the abdominal cavity; involved in the processing of blood toxins, glucose metabolism, and the digestion of food.

low anterior resection: Major operation performed to treat rectal cancer.

lymph nodes: Pea-size glands located throughout the body and involved in fighting off infection.

Lynch syndrome: A rare inherited condition that increases your risk of colon and other cancers.

M

magnetic resonance imaging (MRI) scan: A specialized X-ray test using electrons to create detailed pictures of the human body.

malignant tumor: A tumor that is cancerous and can spread to other parts of the body.

metastasis: The spreading of a cancerous growth to organs in the body.

minimally invasive surgery: Surgery performed using small incisions, fiber-optic cameras, and small surgical instruments.

mucosa: The inner layer of cells lining an organ.

muscularis propria: The muscle layer of cells surrounding the mucosa in an organ.

mutation: A DNA change in a gene resulting in an abnormal functioning and, potentially, disease.

N

nadir: The point at which blood cell counts are at their lowest point after chemotherapy treatment.

nasogastric tube: A long, clear plastic tube inserted into a patient's stomach during and after surgery to drain any fluid collecting in the stomach.

neoadjuvant chemotherapy: Chemotherapy that is given before the primary or main treatment.

neuropathy: A disease or abnormality of the nervous system.

neutropenia: Describes the state of a very low white blood cell count.

O

oncologist: A doctor specializing in the medical treatment of cancer.

P

palliative treatment: Treatment aimed at slowing a disease rather than curing it.

pathologist: A doctor trained specifically to examine tissue and perform autopsies.

patient-controlled anesthesia (PCA): A type of postoperative pain control involving the continuous infusion of intravenous narcotic medicine.

pelvic exenteration: A radical surgical treatment that removes all organs from the pelvic cavity. The urinary bladder, urethra, rectum, and anus are removed.

pericolonic fat: The fat immediately adjacent to the colon wall.

Peutz-Jeghers syndrome: An inherited disease resulting in the formation of numerous benign colorectal polyps at an early age.

polyp: An abnormal growth that can occur in any organ, especially the colon. Polyps can be benign or malignant.

port: A small medical appliance that is installed beneath the skin. A catheter connects the port to a vein. Under the skin, the port has a septum through which chemotherapy drugs can be injected.

positron emission tomography (PET) scan: An imaging test that shows how tissues and organs are functioning

R

radiation oncologist: A doctor trained to perform radiation therapy on patients for the treatment of cancer.

radiofrequency ablation: A medical procedure in which a tumor is removed using heat generated from the high frequency alternated current.

radiologist: A doctor trained to perform and read all X-rays.

rectum: The last six to ten inches of colon leading to the anus.

recurrence: The return of a cancer during the follow-up period after the initial treatment has been carried out.

red blood cells: Cells circulating in the body involved in the metabolism of oxygen and iron.

resection: To remove surgically.

S

screening: Periodic testing for a specific disease.

serosa: The outer layer of cells surrounding any organ.

sessile: Describes the shape of a polyp as being flat and broad based.

sigmoid colon: The part of the colon starting at the end of the left, or descending, colon and connecting to the rectum.

sigmoidoscopy: A procedure using a lighted scope to examine the sigmoid colon and rectum.

snare: A wire device used to remove polyps from the colon during a colonoscopy.

spleen: The organ located beneath the left rib cage and involved in the immune system's ability to fight infection.

staging: The process of classifying the extent to which a diagnosed cancer has spread.

stoma: A surgically created opening in the large intestine that allows the passage of feces into a pouch or other collection device.

stomatitis: Inflammation of the mucous lining of any of the structures in the mouth.

stool DNA test: Designed to identify recognizable DNA markers in cells that are continually shed from the lining of the colon and into stool.

submucosa: The layer of cells just beneath the inner lining, or mucosa, of an organ.

subtotal colectomy: An operation involving removal of 90 percent of the colon.

T

targeted therapy: Therapy that mainly attacks the cancer cells and does not affect normal cells. This generally means milder side effects compared to those resulting from chemotherapy.

Glossary

tenesmus: The sensation of pressure in the rectum immediately after having a bowel movement.

three-dimensional conformal radiation therapy (3D-CRT): Treatment that uses computers and special imaging techniques to show the size, shape and location of a tumor.

thrombocytopenia: Any disorder in which there is an abnormally low amount of platelets.

total colectomy: An operation performed to remove the entire colon.

transanal excision: Surgery for rectal cancer that spares the anus and leaves the sphincter intact.

transrectal ultrasound: An imaging test using sound waves to evaluate a tumor in the rectum.

transverse colon: The portion of the colon connecting the right and left colon segments.

tubular: Referring to the tubelike shape of cells in some polyps.

tubulovillous: A type of polyp that grows in the colon and other places in the gastrointestinal tract and sometimes in other parts of the body.

tumor: A tissue growth that can be benign or malignant.

tumor markers: Substances found in the blood, urine, or body tissues that can be elevated if caner is present.

Turcot syndrome: An inherited disease resulting in the formation of numerous colorectal polyps.

U

ulcerative colitis: A serious chronic inflammatory disease of the large intestine and rectum characterized by recurrent episodes of abdominal pain, fever, chills, and profuse diarrhea.

ultrasound test: An X-ray or imaging test using sound waves to analyze an organ.

V

villous: Refers to the microscopic description of a particular polyp.

virtual colonoscopy: A medical imaging procedure that uses X-rays and computers to produce two- and three-dimensional images of the colon from the lowest part, the rectum, all the way to the lower end of the small intestine.

Index

A

abdomen, 38, 39
abdomen lining, 84
abdominal cavity, 3, 31
abdominal cramping, 10, 67, 90, 97
abdominal pain, 15, 18, 54
    chronic, 9
abnormal blood tests, 25
abnormal heart rhythms, 51
acneiform rash, 75
acute neuropathy, 70
acute renal failure, 76
adenocarcinoma, 7
adjuvant therapy, 61
adrenal glands, 81
age as a risk factor, 14, 61
Agency for Toxic Substances and Disease Registry (ATSDR), 16
alcohol, 104
allergic reaction, 75, 76
ambulatory infusion pump, 64, 65
American Cancer Society, 1, 2, 16
anal sphincter, preservation, 61

anemia, 9, 19, 24, 72
    causes, 25
anesthesiologist, 47
antibiotics, 71, 75
antinausea mediations, 63, 68
antioxidants, 103, 104
anus, 2, 3, 4, 22
anxiety, 28
appendix, 3
appetite changes, 9, 19, 28, 89, 97
areas to which colorectal cancer can spread, 31
asbestos exposure as a risk factor, 16
ascending colon, 3
aspirin, 105

B

bacteremia, 11
    symptoms, 11
bacteria, 80
bacterial infection, 11
barium, 24
barium enema, 21, 24
benign cancer cells, 33
biopsy, 20, 30, 47, 102

support groups, 29, 54, 58
suppositories, 91
surgery, 37, 38–59
  complications, 45, 46
surgical removal of rectum, 44
surgical site infections, 46

T
targeted therapy, 78, 79
  candidates for, 78
  effectiveness, 79
  side effects, 79
temporary colostomy, 55
tenesmus, 9
thinking impairment, 77
three-dimensional conformal
  radiation therapy (3D-CRT),
  86
thrombocytopenia, 73
thyroid gland, 13, 81
tissue margins, 42
tissue samples, 66
TNM classification system, 37
topical gels, 75
total blood volume, 24
total colectomy, 43
transducer, 27
transanal excision, 44
transfusions, 51, 73
transrectal ultrasound (TRUS),
  27
transverse colectomy, 41
transverse colon, 3
treatment plans, 28, 30, 37
tubulovillous precancerous
  polyps, 6
tubular precancerous polyps,
  6

tumor, 66
  mapping, 86
  proteins, 66
  treatments to shrink, 61, 85
tumor cells, 32
tumor markers, 94, 95
tumor samples, 30
Turcot syndrome, 13
type of cancer cells present,
  32, 33

U
ulcerative colitis, 5, 15, 20, 95,
  102
  causes, 15
  recurrence, 15
ultrasound testing, 27
unintended weight loss, 9, 11

V
vaccines, 80
villous precancerous polyps, 6
virtual colonoscopy, 23
viruses, 66, 80
vital signs, 48
vomiting, 21, 54, 68, 69

W
waste product, 2
weight loss, 9, 11, 18, 28, 97
well-differentiated cells, 33
Western diet, 14
wheezing, 75
white blood cell count, 65, 71,
  92
white blood cells, 65, 66, 71,
  92
wound infection, 53

X
X-rays, 24, 25, 27, 28, 87

ABOUT THE AUTHORS

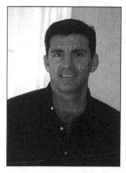 **Paul Ruggieri, M.D.,** is a board-certified general surgeon in private practice in southeastern Massachusetts. Dr. Ruggieri received his medical degree from the Georgetown University School of Medicine in Washington, D.C. Dr. Ruggieri completed his surgical internship and residency at Barnes Jewish Hospital, Washington University School of Medicine, St. Louis, Missouri.

After his medical training, Dr. Ruggieri joined the Army and was stationed at the U.S. Army hospital in Fort Polk, Louisiana. During his time in the military, he rose to the rank of major, received the Army Commendation and Meritorious Service medals, and became the chief of the department of surgery. In 1995, Dr. Ruggieri entered a private surgical practice near Nashville, Tennessee. In 1998, he returned to his native New England to join a surgical group in southeastern Massachusetts.

Dr. Ruggieri is a fellow in the American College of Surgeons and is a member of the Society of American Gastrointestinal Endoscopic Surgeons. He is also the co-author of *A Simple Guide to Thyroid Disorders* (Addicus Books, 2010) and is the author of *The Surgery Handbook: A Guide to Understanding Your Operation* (Addicus Books, 1999). He also authored *Confessions of a Surgeon* (Berkley, 2012) and *The Cost of Cutting* (Berkley, 2014).

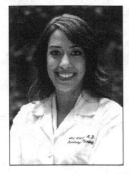

Arti A. Lakhani, M.D., is board certified in the fields of internal medicine, hematology, and oncology, and currently works in the Chicagoland area. Dr. Lakhani received her medical degree and completed her residency at Rush University in Chicago and her hematology/oncology fellowship at Loyola University in Maywood, IL. She has published numerous articles in the fields of hematology and oncology, and is dedicated to caring for patients with complex malignancies. She has also completed a fellowship in integrative medicine and has established an Integrative Oncology Center to serve the needs of the surrounding community.

Dr. Lakhani is a member of the American Society of Clinical Oncology, the American Society of Hematology, and the Society of Integrative Oncology. Her mission is to provide cancer patients with state-of-the-art treatments while incorporating evidence-based complementary and alternative methods. She defines integrative oncology as a practice that not only treats disease, but aims to prevent cancer recurrence, reduce side effects, improve quality of life, and most importantly empower the patient to take an active role in their personal health.

Consumer Health Titles from Addicus Books

Visit our online catalog at www.AddicusBooks.com

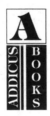